THE WELLNESS BLUEPRINT

The Complete Mind/Body Approach to Reclaiming Your Health & Wellness

DR. MAIYSHA CLAIRBORNE, M.D.

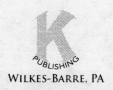

WILKES-BARRE, PA

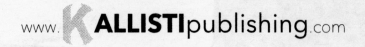

www.**K**ALLISTIpublishing.com

332 Center Street • Wilkes-Barre, PA 18702

Any errors, typographical or otherwise, are here for a purpose: some people actually enjoy looking for them and we strive to please as many people as possible. If you should find any erros, please contact us via our web site. We'll make a the correction for future editions—and maybe reward you with a small gift.

This book is not intended as a substitute for the medical advice of physicians. The reader should regularly consult a physician in matters relating to his/her health and particularly with respect to any symptoms that may require diagnosis or medical attention.

ISBN-13 978-0-9848162-2-4

Library of Congress Control Number: 2012945662

DESIGNED & PRINTED IN THE UNITED STATES OF AMERICA

TABLE OF CONTENTS

I dedicate this book to my baby boy, Delsyn...
Through all my years of practicing medicine, wellness,
spirituality, and yoga, you have been my best teacher so far!
Through you I truly have experienced unconditional love and
patience. You have trained me even more rigorously in
self-care, self-responsibility, and loving boundaries.
Because of you, I am more open and vulnerable—and I
experience intimacy to new levels. You have taught me the
importance of asking for help from my community and those
who love me most.
You have reminded me of how much my people really do love
me and how willing—no! excited—they are to support me
when I actually have the courage ask and am open to receive.
Through you I have learned to communicate more
authentically and effectively. Through you I have experienced
the deepest possible spiritual connection.
Finally, it is through you, my baby boy Delsyn, that I have
come to know my own strength and tenacity.
I love you, my darling son!
Thank you for teaching me the best lessons before coming out
of the womb!

FOREWORD

BY DR. MANONMANI ANTONY

THERE IS AN ADAGE THAT YOU MAY HAVE HEARD: "When you have your health, you have everything. When you do not have your health, nothing else matters at all."

That quote is attributed to Augusten Burroughs. Regardless of who said it, nothing is more true. You can be wealthy. You can be beautiful. You can be famous. Without your health, none of that matters.

I see that every day in my practice. I am a pain relief physician and the owner of the Sussex Pain Relief Center in Bedford, Delaware.

I've seen young men in the prime of their life unable to perform the simplest of tasks because of pain.

I've seen mothers unable to coddle their babies because of ill health.

I've seen ambitious people unable to work because their health would not allow it.

Money didn't matter. Not even love mattered. Without their health and wellness they had nothing.

My patients who became better and who, with proper care and treatment, went on to have active and full lives had two things.

The first was hope. They carried with them the idea

and attitude that things would get better — that they would become better. Hope got them through the tough times.

The second thing they had — the one I would consider more important and instrumental in their recovery — was the willingness, if not the outright audacity, to reclaim their health and wellness. These people not only acted on my advice, the advice of their physician, they aggressively pursued healthy practices, constructive attitudes, and anything and everything that would help them on their journey.

Without knowing it, they followed much of what Dr. Maiysha Clairborne writes in this book, *The Wellness Blueprint*.

Beyond my patients, the healthy and well people I know — friends, family, associates, and even myself — practice these methods in one form or another. We know that a person's health is only as good as how one cares for oneself. Much like a car, with proper care and maintenance, it will last a long time; without care, the car is prone to break and, eventually, not work.

The doctor-patient relationship is a very symbiotic one. Yes, a doctor can do many amazing things for you — things that you could not do for yourself. A doctor cannot force you to take his or her advice or to follow his or her instructions.

More importantly, a doctor cannot force nor cajole you into taking your daily health and wellness into your own hands. As we are seeing and hearing more frequently, preventative care is taking precedence over critical care. What that means is that it is of paramount importance now more than ever for a person — for you — to practice healthy habits and hold healthy attitudes on a daily basis rather than waiting for an emergency situation to force you to do so.

Sadly, we don't see people doing that all too often. For that, there is no excuse. As Dr. Clairborne will illustrate to you in this book, adopting such practices and methods is not difficult. On the contrary, not many things are easier.

Another adage, this one from the esteemed Benjamin Franklin, is "An ounce of prevention is worth a pound of cure." Why wait until you are reminded of the value of good health and wellness to take care of yourself? Why wait for your doctor's warning about high blood pressure or eating unhealthy foods before you take the reins of your own health?

Dr. Clairborne has written a life-changing book with The Wellness Blueprint. It's applications are unlimited — there isn't a patient of any issue or circumstance who could not be helped by this book. It's results can prove to be nothing short of amazing. It's one of those books that come along every few years that can — and hopefully will — impact how health and wellness is viewed.

To my fellow physicians and practitioners, I urge you to peruse this book and to take as many of the ideas and methods you find and put them into use in your practice. Only as we doctors approach our patients from the perspective of the body, mind, and soul (however you wish to define that) will we see our patients understand the value of their health and the improvements that come with that understanding. Is doing this as simple as prescribing a medication and telling the patient to "take two and call him in the morning"? Of course not. The rewards, though, are greater. The benefits to both you and your patient are broader and long-lasting. The value, as you will discover, is simply priceless.

Dr. Maiysha Clairborne will help you reclaim and put together your health and wellness with her *Wellness Blueprint*. Take advantage of what she has to offer. While it may or may not be a matter life and death, it is a matter of having "everything" and having "nothing."

Dr. Manonmani Antony, M.D.
Sussex Pain Relief Center
July, 2014

PREFACE

EVERYONE KNOWS THAT THEY SHOULD LIVE healthier. Whether it's the idea that they should eat better or exercise or any of the myriad ways that one defines "healthy," people—including you—know that you *should* be doing things better.

That's all well and good. There's only one problem: that one, single, small word—"should."

We know what we should do. The problem is that we don't know how to go about actually doing it. "I should eat better," all of us have said at one time or another. The problem is that we don't know exactly what that means (become a vegetarian? more salads? is fish good nowadays?) nor do we know how to go about it (who has the time to prepare meals? can I use the microwave? am I still allowed to have a cheeseburger?)

Even the idea of exercise becomes perplexing when faced with actually doing it: Is a gym membership necessary? Do I need a weight set? Do I have to awaken at dawn and train like Rocky?

Yes, here are hundreds (at least) of complicated programs and so-called "self-help secrets" out there that you can buy or join. There are books written on everything from how to "make yourself over" to how to lose weight. The truth is that while some of these books and programs have valid concepts and methods, few have a simplicity that can be immediately practiced during a busy day at work or in the midst of a stressful situation. In other words, far too many of these concepts are difficult to integrate into daily life. Thus, the point of them is lost.

So how is this book that you hold in your hands, *The Wellness Blueprint*, different?

The Wellness Blueprint will guide you to reclaiming your health and wellness by deconstructing a healthy lifestyle into simple steps that can be integrated easily—and often immediately—into your daily life. You will find easy-to-remember exercises that you can do at practically any time anywhere you are. You will find tools to reduce stress, to bring about better relationships, and to foster improved healing.

In short, you will find a plan—a blueprint—for having and living a healthy life.

One of my mottoes is "Small action steps lead to big changes that will ultimately improve your quality life." Some small changes can lead to big consequences. You're going to see how many times a simple smile can do everything from reducing stress to contribute to a happier workplace. You'll discover a method of getting rid of a headache—even a migraine!—that doesn't require pills or potions or secluding yourself from everything and everyone. You'll learn simple words and phrases that can bring about greater bonding and love in your relationships.

All of this and more is part of this plan, this blueprint.

You know what you want. *The Wellness Blueprint* is here to let you know not only what you should do, but also how to go about doing it. I'm a firm believer in the K.I.S.S. philosophy. For those who don't know, that means "Keep It Simple, Sweetie." In all my years studying and practicing medicine, from medical school to my residency to my practice, what I've encountered more than anything is not an unwillingness on my patients' parts to get healthy, rather it was a habit of making things too complex.

Well, the good news is that it doesn't have to be complex. Actually, you'll find that it is not complex at all. Being healthy and well—reclaiming that health and wellness—is simple. If you know what to do. And that's why I'm here and you're reading this book.

I encourage you as you read this book to actually do the exercises, to be a participant in the book. Yes, I know that we like to grab a book and read it before we fall asleep. Take this book in a different manner: choose a time every day where you'll read a few pages—a section, a chapter, whatever your time allows—and actually do the written and mental exercises. Then, as you learn these simple tools and techniques, incorporate them into your daily life. These efforts might be small ("small steps"), yet they will lead to big changes ("giant leaps").

One more aphorism before you begin your journey: I am fond of saying that ultimately, "you get what you give." If you approach someone with a fist, chances are you'll get a fist in return. Likewise, if you approach with a smile, you'll probably get a smile back at you. With this book—with this blueprint you are about to discover and develop—you will only get from it what you put into it.

If you read the entire book and even do all the exercises, yet you don't put into daily practice anything, then you'll find that, for the most part, nothing will change. If you do participate, though, I can guarantee that you will see changes—good changes. Perhaps even surprising changes. It all comes down to you, though. I can supply the ideas and methods and tools; only you can make the choice to use them.

INTRODUCTION
WHAT IS WELLNESS REALLY?

WELLNESS IS A HOT TOPIC OF DISCUSSION RIGHT now. From the Affordable Care Act to healthy lunches in schools to pharmaceutical companies' deeds and misdeeds, we hear about health and wellness on the news, at the dinner table, and around the water cooler.

So many people are joining the bandwagon with detoxification and cleansing, colonics, exercise, weight-loss programs, herbal therapies, and homeopathy—all claiming to be well. However, even with all of these natural modalities, we are (as a society) missing very important steps.

That leads to the question: *What is wellness?* What does it really mean? What is this "wellness" that is on the lips of everyone from the president to the man on the street?

As defined, wellness is not just the absence of disease; it's a complete state of mental, physical, and social well-being that allows for a better quality of life. What we see in our state of health from day-to-day is only the tip of the iceberg. The underlying causes of preventable disease rest deep below the surface in basic endeavors such as lifestyle, stress management, and mental health. When these are not addressed or are practiced poorly, major illnesses will almost inevitably occur.

A key concept in wellness is that our well-being is reflected in the energy we take in versus the energy we put out. I saw this clearly reflected when I was in my residency program. Patients would come into the office strictly wanting to deal with what was physically wrong with them. What I began to notice is that no matter how physically well a patient was, if their mental or emotional well-being was out of place they still manifested illness. Conversely, I also noticed that patients with seemingly severe illnesses who had a more balanced state of mind and lifestyle—they incorporated spirituality, play, and had a strong community support system—tended to do very well (had a higher quality of life) despite their illness. That simple observation highlighted to me the difference between health and well-being.

I also noticed, both as I was studying in medical school and continuing to this very day, that most of my colleagues were focused more on "fixing" patients and putting out "fires" rather than preventing them. It didn't—and doesn't—make sense to me to wait until a patient is ill before we began to look at their illness. It also doesn't make sense to me to simply tell a patient to "go eat better and be more relaxed" when we know good and well that they don't know the least bit of what to do once they leave the doctor's office.

This is one of the main reasons I started my practice. I am committed empowering and teaching that being well is more than just being physically healthy. Well-being includes mental, emotional, spiritual, and social facets.

Let's just look at the facts for a minute. There is plenty of research that shows the relationship between emotional well-being and physical well-being. Furthermore, there is research that shows that healthy relationships impact emotional well-being. So let's take relationships as an example. Medical studies show that

Δ   people who have strong social networks tend to live longer[1];

Δ   the heart rate and blood pressure of people with healthy relationships respond better to stress[2];

Δ   healthy relationships are associated with healthier hormone function and enhanced immune system[3];

Δ   and people with healthy relationships have a greater ability to fight off infectious disease[4].

Furthermore, a recent study (published in May 2012) in the issue of *NeuroImage* suggests that one effect of the

1   Berkman, L.F. (1995). The role of social relations in health promotion. Psychosomatic Medicine, 57, 245-254.

2   Broadwell, S.D., Light, K.C. (1999). Family support, and cardiovascular responses in married couples during conflict and other interactions. Int J Behav Med, 6, 40-63.

3   Seeman, T.E., Berkman, L.F., Blazer, D., Rowe, J.W. (1994). Social ties and support and neuroendocrine functions: The MacArthur studies of successful aging. Annals of Behavioral Medicine, 16, 95-106.

Uchico, B.N., Cacioppo, J.T., Kiecolt-Glaser, J.K. (1996). The relationship between social support and physiological processes: A review with emphasis on underlying mechanism and implications for health. Psychological Bulletin, 119, 448-531.

4   Cohen, S., Doyle, W.J., Skoner, D.P., Rabin, B.S., Gwaltney, J.M. Jr (1997). Social ties and susceptibility to the common cold. Journal of American Medical Association, 277, 1940-44.

Cohen, S., Gottlieb, B.H., Underwood L. (2000). Social relationships and health. In Cohen, S., Underwood, L. & Gottlieb, B.H. (Eds), Social Support Measurement and Interventions: A Guide for Health and Social Scientists. New York: Oxborg University Press.

practice of mindfulness is increased brain connectivity. Researchers at UCLA compared the brain activity of volunteers who had finished eight weeks of mindfulness-based stress reduction training with that of volunteers who did no such training. Functional MRI scans showed enhanced connections in several regions of the volunteers' brains who completed the mindfulness-based stress reduction training. Similar studies have been done at Massachusetts General Hospital.

Are you beginning to get the picture? Wellness is more than just physical health. So what is this book about? In my experience, many people know what they should do, but don't always know the pathway—or even the starting point. This book is a practical guide to achieving and maintaining a structure that creates workability in the lives of even the busiest people. My commitment is that people live a life they love and live it powerfully. This book is the blueprint to that life.

This book is divided into four parts. The first part is the Foundation and deals with taking responsibility for one's health and wellness. The second part is the Floorplan and is where we will delve into specific techniques for building that mind-body connection. The third part, the Structure, will detail how you can develop a life—and a lifestyle—that encourages your continued health and wellness. Finally, the fourth part, Pathways, will provide you with tools to take you both deeper as well as beyond what you discover in *The Wellness Blueprint*. Throughout the book, we will go into specific areas of life such as nutrition, your emotional and mental states, communication, work-play balance, intimacy, and spirituality. As we look at each specific area, you will find specific exercises and tips that you can start using immediately in your life. What you can expect to see as a result of implementing these practices into your daily life will be increased energy and focus, better relationships at work and home, more fun and laughter on a daily basis, a deeper sense of connectedness, and an overall peace of mind.

In short, you will reclaim your health and wellness and, in doing so, enjoy a higher quality of life.

It was the poet Virgil who wrote that "the greatest wealth is health." Without health, without wellness, a person can have all the riches and all the fame in the world—and it would be as if they had nothing. If you're reasonably healthy now, then your life is going to become better as you enjoy newfound energy and focus. If you're dealing with a health issue, you're going to discover ways to reclaim the health and wellness you deserve. Even if you suffer from a chronic condition, you're going to be illuminated to ways and means that will make your life more than livable—you'll actually find enjoyment and peace.

So, join me and begin building a life of health and wellness. Here's the Blueprint. It's only up to you to **Change your mind—Shift Your Heart—Transform Your Life**.

Dr. Maiysha Clairborne, M.D.
March, 2014

THE
WELLNESS
BLUEPRINT

"Autobiography in Five Short Chapters" by Portia Nelson

I

I walk down the street.
There is a deep hole in the
sidewalk.
I fall in.
I am lost ... I am helpless.
It isn't my fault.
It takes me forever to find
a way out.

II

I walk down the same
street.
There is a deep hole in the
sidewalk.
I pretend I don't see it.
I fall in again.
I can't believe I am in the
same place.
But it isn't my fault.
It still takes a long time to
get out.

III

I walk down the same
street.
There is a deep hole in the
sidewalk.
I see it is there.
I still fall in ... it's a habit.
My eyes are open.
I know where I am.
It is my fault.
I get out immediately.

IV

I walk down the same
street.
There is a deep hole in the
sidewalk.
I walk around it.

V

I walk down another street.

PART I

FOUNDATION

To keep the body in good health is a duty, otherwise we shall not be able to keep our mind strong and clear.

—**Buddha**

1
THE DIFFERENT ASPECTS OF WELLNESS
LAYING YOUR WELLNESS FOUNDATION

WHAT DO YOU THINK WHEN YOU HEAR THE WORD "wellness"? Nutrition and fitness? Doctors and health care professionals? Remedies and cures? Perhaps you think just feeling fine and being in "good health."

When you take into account everything that wellness encompasses, you discover that it is not just eating right, exercising, or the various modes of healthcare. It's not something that only takes place in the doctor's office or operating room. It's not a pill that you take.

When contemplating wellness, you find that it is something that is right here and right now. Most importantly, it's something that *is* within your control. It's something that you can claim (or *re*claim) and with it improve your life dramatically.

In this book, we will explore the different aspects of wellness that most doctors or other health practitioners often overlook and that can have a significant impact on your day-to-day life. You will explore the main areas of life that affect your overall wellbeing as well as learn techniques that you can immediately apply.

It's a journey that you and I will make one step at a time. In doing so, we will make a blueprint from which you can craft your wellness—a wellness that you will own and that will impact every aspect of your life.

Let's begin by building a good foundation upon which you will develop your wellness. Like the foundation of a sturdy house, this wellness foundation will support everything that you do to claim and improve your wellbeing.

This foundation consists of your two different modes (or states) and the different aspects of wellness that contribute to your wellness. These ideas will aid you as you transition into a state of wellness and is an important first step in your blueprint for wellness.

LEARNING AND PROTECTING MODES

When you are absorbing and processing information, you will be in one of two modes: **learning mode** or **protecting mode**.

Learning mode is a relaxed or "centered" state. When you are in learning mode, you tend to be more curious, open, expansive, creative, understanding, and forgiving.

You feel good when you are in learning mode. You feel relaxed. Your breathing is slow and steady. You feel accepted and at peace. Your body loses tension and your heart beats at a gentle pace. Overall, you feel a sense of openness.

Protecting mode is a tense state. When you are in protecting mode, you tend to be more defensive, judgmental, fearful, numb, anxious, shameful, and shut down.

It's easy to tell when you are in a protecting mode because it doesn't feel good to you. Your heart races. You can feel your chest tighten and your head may ache. You become fatigued. Your muscles become tense, which leads to frowning and foot tapping. Overall, you feel a sense of denial and of being closed to everyone and everything around you.

I'm certain that you've felt both of those states. We all have. There are times when things just seem "right" in the world to us and times when they just don't.

Obviously, being in learning mode is far better than being in protecting mode, but we can't be in learning mode constantly. It's just not humanly possible.

The key, though, is to *notice* when you are in protecting mode so that you can shift yourself back to learning mode. You accomplish this by consciously relaxing and centering yourself. Take a few deep breaths and become aware of the physical sensations in your body. Gently bring yourself into learning mode, feeling an easier and deeper breathing pattern and more relaxed mental and physical state. (As you progress through this book, you will learn techniques for you to do this. The important thing now is to at the very least notice when you are in protecting mode.) If you are unable to make that shift, then it may be a good time to stop whatever activity you are doing and return to it later. Trying to force yourself into learning mode when you are physically and mentally unable is just not productive for anyone.

Throughout this book, it will be beneficial for you to stop and check-in with yourself to see whether you are currently in learning or protecting mode. Begin right now:

Where are you now? How is your body feeling? Take thirty seconds to reflect on what learning mode or protecting mode feels like to you. As you'll see as you progress, doing this will prove to be very beneficial and will soon become almost second-nature to you.

THE DIMENSIONS OF WELLNESS

When looking at total well-being, I refer to a system developed by Dr. John Travis called the "Wellness Energy System." In this system, your body intakes and expends energy in sixteen different ways, which he calls "dimensions." Think of this process like water running through a pipe: something goes in and something goes out. This is the foundation of your wellness system.

Your **energy intakes** are:

Breathing   Eating   Smell   Sight   Hearing
Touch   Taste

Your **energy expenditures** are the following:

Feelings   Movement   Communication
Thinking   Working   Playing
Relationships   Finding Your Life Purpose
Spiritual Interaction

As core supports of Dr. Travis' Wellness Energy System—and, by extension, your own wellness blueprint—are **self-responsibility** and **self-love**, as they allow all the other aspects to flow together.

Self-responsibility refers to the idea that only you can truly know yourself and therefore only you are responsible for getting what you need in order to be well. You practice self-responsibility by knowing yourself and realizing your needs and expressing yourself to other people effectively.

Self-love is the notion that you should realize and embrace your uniqueness as well as hold yourself as your own best friend. As you do this, you will come to understand that you are connected with all things.

Actions within this wellness energy system create a cellular imprint, a veritable impression on your physical being. The imprint can be shifted and changed over time as you change your behavior. As you create these impressions within the wellness energy system, your body strives for "homeostasis," or balance.

As with a financial budget, if there is too much discrepancy between the intake and expenditure, your body falls out of balance. The end result is mental, emotional, and/or physical disease.

Let's look at how this can happen in real life.

Anita's Discrepancy (Example)

Anita has been feeling very anxious lately due to recent layoffs at work. She is a single mother of one child from her first marriage and has a new boyfriend. Normally, Anita eats a well-balanced diet and manages to exercise three times a week. Because she's been obsessing about being laid off, she hasn't been able to sleep and is too tired to cook or go to the gym, so she starts picking up fast food on her way home. Due to these changes, Anita gains weight. She now looks in the mirror and is not happy with what she sees. She scolds herself, telling herself that if she doesn't lose this weight, her boyfriend will leave her. This creates even more anxiety and she begins to distance herself from her boyfriend. He becomes confused and wonders why she has become less interested. Anita even becomes short and easily irritated with her son, with whom she was usually patient and understanding. At work, Anita loses her edge, becoming easily distracted and never seeming to get anything done.

Eventually, Anita realizes that this fear is affecting her in all aspects of her life and she consults with a doctor who recommends that she try deep breathing exercises, even a meditation or a yoga class. Anita takes his advice and, after two weeks in a meditation class, begins to feel better. She begins to find time to work out again. She begins eating healthy and reconnecting with her significant other.

See how the imbalance in just her feeling (anxiety due to the layoffs at work) and thinking (worrying about being laid off herself) dimensions threw the other areas (weight, exercise, relationships, and work) off?

Because Anita was feeling anxious, she was not able to sleep, which caused her to be too tired to exercise or cook. Her eating habits became unhealthy and she gained weight. Her self-love, as a result, went down and her self-image became negative. This affected how she related to her boyfriend. These feelings overflowed onto her son and even affected her performance at work.

This example highlights the importance of finding

balance in our lives within these twelve areas of wellness. Just one errant aspect can create a domino effect that will impact many areas of your life.

TAKING INVENTORY OF OUR ASPECTS

To discover whether we are in balance or out of balance, we take an inventory of our wellness aspects. We look at a specific behavior, thought, or action and see how it affects each area of wellness. This can also be done the other way around by looking at how the balance of the wellness dimensions affects a specific behavior or thought pattern. You can even look at how the dimensions affect each other.

Here's an example.

My fear of failure causes my self-responsibility to be elevated, causing me to over-commit.

My fear of success causes my self-love to be decreased.

My fear of failure causes my thinking to be more negative.

My fear of success causes my communications to be meeker.

Notice how I took a belief—fear of success or fear of failure—and inserted it into each of the twelve dimensions to see how my fear of success (or failure) could affect my sense of wellbeing? That's what you'll do with all of the aspects and all areas of your life.

These are called **spins** and there are five of them.

A *behavior spin*, in which we look at how a behavior is affecting each of these areas.

A *stress spin*, where we look at the stressors.

A *life audit spin*, which determines where we are in relation to these different dimensions.

An *action step spin*, which gives you an idea of how your action steps may affect these twelve areas.

An *attitude spin*, which deals specifically with your feelings, beliefs or thought processes and how they affect these different areas of life.

Take a few minutes now and perform an inventory on yourself. Get a notebook for yourself. In a column, write each of the twelve aspects. Ask yourself how each aspect is in your life and write your answer next to that aspect. Examine some of the effects in your life and ask yourself what might be out of balance.

This information will tell you which areas would be easiest to change and help you shift towards a healthier, more positive, direction.

Speaking of change, the next chapter is all about how to make change simple, successful, and sustainable.

MY WELLNESS INVENTORY

MY ENERGY INTAKES	
Breathing	
Eating	
Smell	
Sight	
Hearing	
Touch	
Taste	
MY ENERGY EXPENDITURES	
Feelings	
Movement	
Communication	
Thinking	
Working	
Playing	
Relationships	
Life Purpose	
Spiritual Interaction	
MY CORE SUPPORTS	
Self-Responsibility	
Self-Love	

2
THE PROCESS OF CHANGE
DEVELOPING LIFE HABITS

WHAT IS CHANGE? WHY IS IT SO HARD TO START and maintain new and healthy behaviors? By definition, change is the alteration or modification from one state to the next. Change can be either positive or negative in nature. Overall, change is inevitable and you have the power to take responsibility for changes in yourself.[1]

In this chapter, you will learn the stages of change and the process of creating sustainable action steps that will get you to the goals you desire.

A couple questions may come to your mind, though: When is change good? And when is it bad?

GOOD CHANGE, BAD CHANGE

Change is good when it fosters growth, serenity, connection, and healthy interaction with others. Some examples of good changes include a new job, beginning a spiritual program, starting an exercise regimen, purchasing a new house, or even making the decision to set healthy boundaries for yourself. Good changes are not always easy nor are they always comfortable, but they work towards

---

1 It is important to remember that while we can influence others, we cannot change others.

your best interest and highest good in the long run.

When changes are not working for your highest good, they tend to cause stress, anxiety, and sometimes even isolation. Some examples of changes in your life that don't serve your common good are taking on too many projects at home or at work, isolation from friends and family, or engaging in addictive behaviors in order to self-medicate your stress or depression.

Let's take a few moments now to take inventory of your current state with respect to change.

What positive changes have occurred in your life?
What negative changes have occurred in your life?
What positive changes do you think you have to make
in order to improve your lifestyle and wellness?

For example, perhaps you received a promotion at work. That promotion, though, may impel you to take on too much responsibility causing you to spend less time with your family. A positive change might be a way to balance your work demands with your family obligations through effective time management.

Write this inventory down for your reference and to keep track of where you are and where you want to go.

THE PROCESSES OF CHANGE

There are nine processes that your brain moves through in the process of change. The processes begin at the first notion of the change and end with the change being effected. All change that we endeavor to implement is governed by these nine processes.

First is **consciousness raising**. This is when you first

become aware of the self and the problem at hand.

Second is a process called **social liberation**. This is looking at or thinking of new alternatives in your external environment. You're not necessarily doing anything; you're just becoming aware of the alternatives available.

Third, you have an **emotional arousal**, where a dramatic life event (perhaps a personal tragedy, a major revelation, or an external event) makes you aware of the potential change that needs to be made. In other words, something hits you "deep."

After this comes a point of **self-reevaluation** (fourth). This is the part where you look at how the problem affects your life negatively and how your life might be better when the change is made. At this point you're weighing the pros and the cons of making this change.

The fifth process of change is **commitment**, where you accept the fact that it is really time to make this change *and* you accept responsibility for that change. The first step of commitment is very private: you make the commitment to yourself. The second step is more powerful: the public commitment occurs when you tell a friend, a family member, or maybe even announce to a group that you're getting ready to change your behavior. It is at this point that you become accountable for the change.

Sixth is **countering** or **counter-conditioning**, which happens when you become aware and get ready to do the activity that replaces the problem behavior.

After counter-conditioning, comes the seventh process, **environmental control**, where you restructure your environment to support the change. For example, changing the schedule, removing offending substances, or even giving yourself little reminders.

The eighth process of change is **reward**. In this stage, you self-praise or you get praise from others for continuing to engage in the changed behavior. It may not be a conscious reward; it may be more of a kickback from the changed behavior itself, an unexpected side effect of the changed behavior. While the rewards can be intentional or non-intentional, it is important to have some intention of rewarding yourself for making the change and sustaining the change.

Finally, the ninth process of change is to **create helping relationships**. This is having an accountability partner—or accepting assistance from other people like family, friends, or a professional—to help you maintain this behavior change.

Let's go through a real life example of how the process of change may work on a daily basis.

TRACEY'S PROCESS OF CHANGE (EXAMPLE)

Tracey steps on the scale and notices her weight gain. She becomes aware that this is a health risk. (Consciousness-raising) *On TV and in magazines, Tracey sees advertisements for products and methods that give her alternatives to her lifestyle.* (Social liberation) *Tracey goes to the doctor and finds out that she has diabetes, high blood pressure, and high cholesterol and is told that these are the result of her being overweight. For Tracey, this is a turning point because she knows that her grandmother and grandfather died from heart disease as a result of diabetes.* (Emotional arousal) *Over the next week, Tracey reflects on how her obesity has affected her life and how her lifestyle has contributed to her problem. She begins to look at the pros and cons of starting a lifestyle change.* (Self-reevaluation) *Tracey decides that if she wants to live a full life, then she has to do something about her weight. She decides that she wants to lose fifty pounds. She tells her family about her goal.* (Commitment) *Next, Tracey decides to make a plan, which includes her plans for dietary and fitness activity. It takes a combination of mental conditioning and actual practice to recondition her out of the old behavior.* (Countering and counter-conditioning) *To support her change, Tracey changes her schedule so that she can exercise, removes junk food and unhealthy snacks form her home, and puts up little reminders and affirmations to help her to continue to be successful in this change.* (Environmental control) *For every five pounds Tracey loses, she buy herself a new piece of clothing.* (Reward) *Tracey reaches out to a friend who walks with her three times a week and she hires a personal trainer to get her started with her program and to keep her motivated. She also joins and attends a weekly support group.* (Create helping relationships)

See how these processes work? These nine processes of change apply to many other areas of life including beginning or ending relationships, relocation, job or career changes, and even starting a family.

Is there a behavior that you're currently trying to

change? Where are you in this process? Take a moment to think about it and write some notes.

THE STAGES OF CHANGE

The stages of change relate closely to the processes of change. Where the processes refer to the mental activity that accompanies change, the stages refer to the transition into physical action. Later, we will fully integrate the two to give you the full picture.

First we have **pre-contemplation**. You are unaware of the need to change and, in order to move to the next stage, there is usually some type of "wake-up call," such as a doctor's warning.

In **contemplation**, much like self re-evaluation in the processes, you begin thinking about changing and assessing the risks and benefits of the change. This is the stage where you are bringing both your rational and emotional self into play in order to come to a commitment to change.

The **preparation** stage involves setting up the support systems you might need in order to maintain or continue to be successful once you make the change. It involves removing temptation, planning on how the action can be taken, arranging understanding and support from family and friends, finding support groups or professionals, and arranging substitutes for the missed habit, activity, or substance. (Be cautious when substituting so you don't substitute a new problem, like overeating or overspending, for the old.)

The **action** stage is next, which is just that: making the change and practicing the new way of being.

Next comes **maintenance**, or sustaining the new

behavior. Sometimes during this stage, the new change starts becoming a new habit.

Sometimes you will find yourself doing what's called **recycling**. This is commonly called "backsliding" and happens when a person relapses back to one of the former stages. Although this is quite common, it's usually where people get discouraged. If recycling occurs, it is important to remember that we are human beings and, as such, not perfect. It is perfectly normal to recycle from time to time. The key is not to consider it a failure, rather look at it as an opportunity to set up more support and better preparation for yourself for when you return to the action stage.

Finally, there is **termination**. This is when the problem has been conquered and the desire to renew the old behavior ceases.[2]

INTEGRATING THE PROCESSES AND STAGES

Let's integrate the processes of change with the stages of change to make the big picture come together.

In each stage of change certain processes happen to move you to the next stage. Thus, within each stage are processes.

In the pre-contemplation stage, you are unaware. Then something happens to raise your consciousness. You are then moved to the contemplative stage, in which emotional arousal occurs about the behavior. You then move to contemplation and self-re-evaluation of changing the

---

2 In some cases, such as lifestyle changes, learning healthy communication, or stress reduction, there is maintenance rather than termination, which involves a certain degree of constant vigilance using tools such as taking things "one day at a time."

behavior happens. This is also where you begin creating helping relationships and you may talk about wanting to change with a friend or a loved one. Once you determine that the benefits of the change outweigh the risks, you move to the preparation stage, which first involves making the commitment to yourself. In this stage you also continue building helping relationships and setting up report systems as well as making plans for the countering behaviors so that you will be prepared to take and sustain action.

Once you feel fully prepared and supported, you begin the action. This includes countering, creating environmental controls, and continuing to utilize the helping relationships that you have built in previous processes. You are also giving yourself rewards for the new behavior.

From then on you are in the maintenance stage. Helping relationships and continued return to consciousness and self-evaluation is key to helping you stay focused on the new behavior or ceasing the old behavior.

Finally, if you are getting rid of the old behavior completely, you arrive at termination. Often, even after termination, if you are ceasing an old, bad habit, it is usually wise to keep helping relationships and environmental controls to prevent recycling, such as with smoking cessation or alcoholism.

Can you think of a specific time or situation where you have applied these principles to a behavior that you have changed? Can you see how you might apply them to a behavior that you are currently attempting to change?

WHAT DO YOU WANT TO CHANGE?

Let's do an exercise to determine what behavior you would like to change. Fill in the blanks of the following sentence:

My ___(behavior)___ *causes my **self-love** to be* _____.

You will repeat this sentence with each of the twelve aspects of wellness. You will do this by copying the sentence and replacing "self-love" with each of the other aspects of wellness[3].

Here are examples of how this sentence may be completed:

My obsessive thinking, stress, and worry causes me to have low self-love.

My obsessive thinking, stress, and worry causes me to be overly responsible.

My obsessive thinking, stress, and worry causes my breathing to be restricted.

With your inventory completed, what have you learned about your behavior? It may even be good to discuss this with someone else.

WHAT STAGE ARE YOU IN?

Write down your answers to the following reflective questions to determine what stage you are currently in.

In what stage of change are you?

If you are in the contemplative stage, what process are

3 To refresh your memory, they are Self-responsibility, Breathing, Sensing, Eating, Feeling, Thinking, Communicating, Moving, Playing, Working, Intimate Relationships or Close Relationships, the Ability to Find Meaning in Life, and Relationship with Your Higher Power.

you aware of that assist you in moving to the next stage? Are you doing a self-evaluation? Are you beginning to set up helping relationships?

If you are in the preparation stage, have you created a plan and set up supports that will help your action steps to be more solid and manageable for maintenance? Have you made a firm commitment to yourself? Have you set up an accountability system, either being accountable to yourself or someone else?

If you are in the action stage, are you continuing to utilize your helping relationships, support systems, to keep you strong and accountable? Are you giving yourself rewards for the good behavior?

If you have moved into the maintenance stage, are you continuing with your helping relationships? Do you continue to re-evaluate your process constantly, and its benefits?

Reflect on your answers before you continue.

RESISTANCE AND EXCUSES

If you are in a pre-contemplative or a contemplative stage and are feeling some physical or emotional resistance to change, know that this is a normal part of the process. We all have resistance at some point, especially at the beginning.

When you encounter resistance, ask yourself these questions. The answers to them will help you get through your resistance and move forward to the next stage.

Where is this resistance coming from?

What excuse am I using?

What benefit or secondary gain am I getting from

this undesired behavior? (Is it attention, emotion comfort, or some type of excitement?)

Remember that excuses are valid. They represent the door to where your resistance is coming from. Here are some example excuses, what they represent, and solutions to overcoming them.

Excuse: I just don't have enough time to exercise.

Translation: I cannot bear the thought of adding one more thing onto my plate. It is just so overwhelming and I wouldn't even know where to fit it.

Solution: Get a wellness coach or a personal trainer to help you figure out simple and easy ways to incorporate efficient, fun, and interesting workouts into your busy lifestyle that don't take away from your work, family, or personal time. It can be done.

Excuse: Eating healthier is so difficult because I have to give up all the things that I love.

Translation: I don't know how to make healthy and tasty snacks. Eating healthy to me seems like it would be boring eating the same things over and over again. I want to be able to enjoy eating like I always have, but I don't know how to do that and be healthy at the same time.

Solution: Take a healthy cooking class. Find healthy, fun recipes online that are quick and easy to prepare.

Excuse: I can't take time for myself. I am so stressed out and I feel stretched thin, but I don't have time in the day to do anything for me. I work long hours, then, when I get home, I have to cook dinner and take care of my children. By the time I'm done it's time to go to bed.

Translation: I am overwhelmed, and I do not know how (or where) to find time for myself.

Solution: Start with small increments of time and build up. Make your lunch break your quiet time. Ask your spouse and children (if they are old enough) for help with household chores that are overwhelming you.

THE DECISIONAL BALANCE SCALE

If you find yourself resisting your new behavior, then do a risk versus benefit assessment. This is called the **Decisional Balance Scale** and it is something that we often do without even realizing it: weighing the pros and the cons.

Take a piece of paper and create two columns. In the first column, write the benefits of keeping the behavior. In the second column, write the risks of keeping the behavior.

Create a second chart like to the one you just used, except in the first column write the benefits of changing the behavior and in the second column write the risks of changing the behavior.

When you are finished, what you will have is an analysis of the pros and the cons of the behavior in question. What you will often find is that if the behavior being weighed is a negative behavior, then the benefits tend to be short-term or visceral benefits while the risks tend to be long-term. Likewise, if the behavior being weighed is positive, then the benefits tend to be long-term while the risks tend to be short-term. To use an easy example, think about smoking: the benefit to keeping the habit is that it feels good (you get a "nic fix") while the risk is that it can (will) eventually kill you.

MY DECISIONAL BALANCE SCALE

KEEPING THE BEHAVIOR

BENEFITS	RISKS

CHANGING THE BEHAVIOR

BENEFITS	RISKS

Keep in mind that this exercise can be done with changing thinking processes, too, and not just actual physical behavior.

Priority

Another factor that can influence your resistance is **priority**. Simply put, is changing the behavior a priority for you? If it is important to you, then you will meet with much less resistance than if it isn't.

Or, perhaps, you have a lot of behaviors that you'd like to change and it is overwhelming and you find yourself not knowing where to start.

A **prioritization grid** is a tool you can use to enumerate what is important to you. Make a chart in which you list the most important things in your life and rate them against the potentially changing behavior. This will help you assess where you are in the process of change and whether you are ready to move to action. If the new behavior is not in your top five priorities, you may need to re-evaluate starting the action, else you may be setting yourself up for the challenge of relapsing or recycling.

Take a moment now to examine your resistances to change. What priority does the new behavior have in your life? Is it in the top five? Top ten? Are you ready for the next step?

If you are ready for the next step, make sure you have the following items ready before you take action.

Your countering behaviors. Remember, you must have new behaviors to replace the old ones in order for you to be successful.

Your helping relationships. These will keep you motivated and accountable.

Your environmental controls. These will help you to avoid temptations and your rewards will keep you motivated to continue the new behavior.

Action Steps

Now you can begin creating action steps.

Action steps are small behaviors that support your ultimate change. Action steps break down your behavior into smaller, more manageable steps so that you can become successful in maintaining that behavior and not become overwhelmed. Action steps are essential because they keep you organized, accountable, and continually moving closer to your new way of living.

There are two guidelines you should observe when you are creating action steps.

Create no more than five action steps at a time. Creating too many action steps can make you overwhelmed, which may lead to an increased risk of recycling. If there are too many action steps at one time, you may become discouraged and anxious, and this makes it more difficult to carry out your action steps with efficiency and confidence.

Make sure your action steps are S.M.A.R.T. Make sure your action steps are **S**pecific, **M**easurable, **A**chievable, **R**ealistic, and **T**ime-bound.

Here is an example of a SMART action step.

Jeanne wants to lose twenty pounds, so she is going to start a new exercise program and an eating program. Her first action step is to begin walking around the

block for thirty minutes three times a week in the af-
ternoon after work, before she cooks dinner.

This action step meets all the SMART criteria. It is very specific and measurable; it is reasonably achievable for Jeanne and realistic; and she puts a time limit on them. Having this SMART action step makes it more likely that Jeanne will follow through.

Now create some action steps of your own.

AN ACTION STEP INVENTORY

Now you are going to take an action step inventory to examine how the action step will affect your twelve areas of wellness. Fill in the blanks of the following sentence.

My (action step) causes my self-love to be _____.

You will take this sentence and replace "self-love" with all of the dimensions of wellness[4]. For example:

My meditation causes me to have more love for myself.
My meditation causes my breathing to be more relaxed.
My meditation causes me to see things brighter.

Now let's move on to examine how your twelve areas of wellness could potentially affect your action step. Fill in the blank of the following sentence.

My self-love causes my (action step) to be _____.

Again, you will copy this sentence and replace "self-love" with the dimensions of wellness. For example,

My breathing causes my morning meditation to be deeper.

CONCLUSION

You have just learned how to identify your process-

4 See Chapter 1, page 4.

es and stages of change as you endeavor to create a new behavior. Remember to be gentle with yourself in this process. We are human and recycling can—and probably will—occur. If this happens, do not give up or get down on yourself. Just get right back into the game by re-evaluating what stage you are in and move forward from there. When you know where you are, it is easier to know where to go. With internal change comes balance, with balance comes healing, and with healing comes improved quality of life.

3
SETTING YOUR INTENTIONS
YOU ARE WHAT YOU BELIEVE

EVER WONDER WHY PEOPLE WHO COMPLAIN ARE always unhappy? Ever wonder why some people can always get what they want? Or why people who say they're always sick are always sick? Or why people who claim to have bad luck usually do? What is the secret to those who never seem to get sick or be stressed? And why is it that one bad mishap can ruin your day?

It's about the power of your **intentions**. In this chapter, we will talk about what keeps people from having the life they want. We will analyze belief systems and understand how they affect your everyday life. We will come to realize the impact of all thought, negative and positive, and you will discover how to overcome the things that holds you back. This chapter will also help you to develop a daily practice that, if done correctly, will change your life.

THE POWER OF INTENTIONS

I'd like to demonstrate the power of intentions with a true story of two women I saw with lupus, a serious autoimmune disease that affects all of the organ systems of the body.

When I was a resident-in-training, one of my regular patients came for a follow-up evaluation. This patient was a lady who had lupus for many years and had been chronically ill ever since. She was constantly having flare-ups, which included pain, lung problems, fatigue, swelling, and she had even been hospitalized several times for stroke and other conditions. She was on disability and when she came in she always talked about how bad she was feeling and how sick she was. I suspect that this had been her mental process for some time before we met—and rightfully so, as her condition was very serious.

At the time of her visit, I evaluated her, treated her to the standard of care for a lupus patient in flare, and scheduled her for a follow-up appointment as usual. At that time, it never occurred to me that her thought and attitude could affect her condition. I was just doing what I had been trained.

Prior to starting my holistic medical practice, I had a patient come in for an evaluation. This woman was a healthy, vibrant young woman, who had also been diagnosed several years with lupus. She stated that while she had not had a flare in a long time, she thought that she might be flaring because she was experiencing some slight joint pain. I began to question her about her condition and its course over the years and she stated that she had never been hospitalized and her flares only occurred during specific times, as she had it under control most other times with diet, activity, and by holding a positive mental attitude. She stated that she was determined not to let this condition take her quality of life. Apparently, her mother and her sister had it as well and they were very healthy as well as very supportive of each other in keeping a positive outlook and, as she said, "keeping it moving."

I was reminded of the other lupus patient, the one from my residency. This young lady reminded me of something that I had already known, but had not truly integrated into my medical practice until that day: *Thoughts are very powerful.*

Why is this story important?

Why do intentions even matter?

They matter because thoughts and words are creative. What you think, what you believe, and what you speak become your reality. You can affect your reception by changing your perception. By changing your pattern of thought, you can affect what comes to you.

THE BLOCKS

What are the things that hold you back from getting what you desire? They are called **blocks** and they are thought patterns and feelings within us that prevent us, both consciously and subconsciously, from acting or becoming that which would be in our best or highest interest.

There are several blocks that impede our progress, but the most common are fear, belief systems, excuses, and self-doubt (which is a derivative of fear).

Fear is one of the single most paralyzing things in life. There are many sources of fear. We will name some of them now, but we will go into more detail on how they affect our self-esteem in the next chapter.

The first type of fear is **instinctive fear,** which is designed to keep you out of danger. Instinctive fear is primal and is necessary to keep us safe. Do you know that feeling you get when you find yourself alone at night in an empty parking garage? That's your instinctive fear kicking in telling you to stay alert.

Next is **fear imposed by statements and actions of family**. This influence usually occurs early on in childhood and sets the basis of how you will view life. While it is true that some fears imposed by family are intended to keep you out of harm's way as well, but many are just carried over from the past experience of someone else. "Don't touch the stove or you'll get burned" or "Don't talk to strangers" are common fears imposed by family. The underlying message of these statements is to inculcate a healthy fear of some of the things that may harm you.

The third type of fear, **fear imposed by statements and actions of colleagues and friends**, comes in the form of discouraging statements from others due to their own past experiences or view of life. They are rarely valid or real. "It's too hard for you to start your own business," "All of my friends died from cancer," "This one doctor didn't even know what the diagnosis was," and "If you go to the chiropractor, he may break your neck" are based on incomplete or false information, but they ingrain a fear that is subconscious, preventing you from taking risk.

Finally, we have **fear that society imposes**. These are fears that can sometimes even cause mass panic, as in the case of the recent swine flu epidemic. Most commonly, though, societally imposed fears are the subtle messages that are perceived to be general "truths" even though they have no basis in fact: "If you are not 'model' skinny, then you are not beautiful," "If you don't have six-pack abs, then you are unattractive," or "The economy is tanking and is only going to get worse." Each of these examples are perceived as true, even though there is no basis for their truthfulness. They are at best constructs of marketing wizards and at worst pessimistic viewpoints of viewer-seeking media outlets. What kind of effects do you think replaying these types of messages has on a society as a whole? On you as a person?

Probably the most powerful fear is **the fear that you impose on yourself**. When you repeatedly tell yourself to be afraid of a particular thing or behavior, it can be challenging to reset and retrain yourself to feel and think differently about that behavior. It *is* possible and you will conquer many of these fears with techniques you will find later in this book. These fears evidence themselves mostly as fear of failure, fear of success, fear of abandonment, or fear of betrayal.

Now that we've talked about fear, let's return to the blocks that impede our progress.

The next one is **clinging to your belief systems**. We live our belief systems like they *are* us. While some belief systems are healthy, there are many fear- and judgment-based belief systems that can hinder you in your wellness journey. Belief systems start from birth. Parents are the first to instill belief systems. Then family members and schools impose their belief systems. Friends and even society impose belief systems. You integrate and continue carrying these beliefs with you throughout your lifetime. Think about the belief systems you carry about yourself and your life. Does your belief system help or hinder you?

Let's pause here and do an exercise. Write down some of your own belief systems regarding the different aspects of wellness (self-love, eating, working, communication, and all the rest). Examine how those beliefs have affected your life. Have they had a positive effect or a negative effect? Have they truly served your best interest in these and other areas of your life? Do you feel that it may be time to explore new belief systems? Remember to stay in learning mode when asking yourself these questions and be as honest as possible with yourself. You may want to refer back to the last chapter on change if you are thinking of exploring new belief systems.

Next, let's move on to **self-doubt**. Self-doubt actually relates both to our fear and our belief systems. Self-doubt works very powerfully on our way of being. When we don't believe in ourselves, we are not motivated to set goals outside of our comfort zone. We will discuss self-doubt more in the next chapter.

Finally, **excuses** are another block that impedes us in our journey to wellness. Excuses are based in fear, self-doubt, and belief systems. While excuses can be valid (as they represent an internal resistance that needs to be addressed), it is easy to excuse yourself right out of opportunities and progress and betterment in all levels in your life. Excuses range from the simple ("I just don't have time to workout.") to the more complex ("I can't eat properly because of the chemotherapy I am undergoing.") While we tend to look at some excuses with a more sympathetic eye, you must keep in mind that an excuse is an excuse and if you truly wish to be better (remember your priorities?) you will let nothing, least of all your excuses based in self-doubt or fear, stop you.

What are some of the excuses you tell yourself that hold you back from doing the things that you know you need to do? What new behavior or project have you been trying to start for weeks or even months? What excuses have you told yourself? What are some of the excuses you use to keep you from pursuing the things that you want? Are these excuses serving your highest good? Make a list so that you can see what is actually happening in your head. Often, seeing is not only believing, it is life-changing.

OVERCOMING THE OBSTACLES

So how do you overcome these obstacles, these blocks?

The simple answer is awareness, acceptance, and action. You can become **aware** of your own self-imposed roadblocks or false roadblocks imposed by others. You can **accept** that they are only roadblocks and that you have a choice—that we all have choices. If you can choose to take a detour, then you choose to take **action** instead. How? Change your thought process. Change your behavior. Set your intentions. Be proactive with your actions and responses rather than reactive. Practice your intentions and new action daily. Remember that while some of these new behaviors may seem overwhelming at first, they come with practice. Finally, it is also important to remember that you do not have to go through it alone. Friends, family, support groups, and even wellness or life coaches are a great way to help keep you accountable and make these steps less scary and more manageable.

INTENTIONS

An **intention** is an anticipated outcome that is planned, or a vision or idea that guides your planned actions. Compare that to the definition of a **goal**: the state of an affair that a plan is intended to achieve.

As you can see, they are very similar words and often they do work together. There is a difference worth noting. Look at the word intention. It begins with the letters *I* and *N*. Now look at the word goal, it begins with the letters *G* and *O*. Use these letters from each word to remember that intention refer to your *internal* meaning, while goals refer to the external, *going* after something.

Now let's look at an example of how goals and intentions work together.

Jeanne desires to lose weight. Her goal is five pounds in 30 days. The intention behind that goal is self-love. From the goal and intentions, she can set a plan of action which includes portion control, an awareness of what she eats, and a plan to exercise at least three times a week for one hour.

A few days into her program, Jeanne does not feel like going to the gym. She tells herself, "You have done so well these last few days, so you can skip a day." At this point,

she remembers her goal of five pounds in thirty days and
the intention of self-love. The goal is in the future. The
intention is in the present moment. She reminded herself
of her goal and intention and now she is empowered, so
she gets up and she gets ready for the gym.

Intentions are not oriented toward a future outcome; rather, intentions are a path of practice that is focused on how you are being in the present moment. So when you set intentions, set them based on understanding what matters most to you and make a commitment to align your actions with your inner values. Remember that setting intentions is a practice because it is an ever-evolving process. Set them and don't forget them! Place them around your home, your car, and your workspace. Live them every day. With intentions, you can reconnect with who you really are inside during emotional storms that cause you to lose touch with yourself. You can then reconnect with your goal and continue taking your steps forward.

Goals help you make your place in the world to become more of an effective person. Intentions provide integrity and unity in your life.

You have five tools at your disposal to help you in setting your intentions correctly. They are Declarations, Visualization, Meditation, Mantras, and Prayer.

DECLARATIONS

Declarations are positive statements of creation in the present tense that create the new possibility of a particular desired outcome. For example, "I love and accept myself as I am," "I have all that I need all of the time,"

"I am the source of creativity and expression," and "I am whole and complete, full of acceptance, love, and joy." Declaring a possibility does not make it happen automatically. The key to realizing the declared goal or possibility is to become what you declare. Following a declaration is a way of being. This brings the intention to reality.

Create your own declarations. Remember that positive statements in the present tense create the possibility of a particular goal or desired outcome. Commit to not only reading this declaration several times on a daily basis but also making your declaration a way of being. Notice how this powerful action shifts your results.

VISUALIZATION

Visualization is the process of creating a mental image in your mind of a particular goal or action that you are trying to achieve. It is used in many areas, such as athletics, business and marketing, and even progressive relaxation. Olympic athletes utilize visualization in their sport and in their training.

The first step in an effective visualization process is becoming relaxed. You can do this through meditation, which will be discussed in more detail in a following chapter. However, the following progressive relaxation technique is a quick way to get relaxed in order to be able to clearly visualize the results that you desire.

PROGRESSIVE RELAXATION TECHNIQUE

Find a comfortable place to sit or lie. As stated earlier, visualization can be used for many different processes or goals, but for the purpose of this book, you will use it for relaxation. Read through the entire exercise first, then try it on your own.

Close your eyes and sit comfortably. Begin to take long, slow, deep breaths, inhaling and exhaling. Notice how your body feels. Begin with your toes and visualize every muscle and tendon in your toes relaxing and releasing.

Now move to the balls of your feet. Feel them relax. Feel them relax and let that relaxation move to your calf muscles. See the muscles lengthening and the neurons slowing their fire, and any muscle spasm completely vanishing.

Let the relaxation next move to your knees. If you feel any pain or inflammation, visualize it. Then visualize a cool, blue light putting out the fire of the inflammation in those joints. Feel the coolness of that blue light and visualize the pain being smothered and then completely disappearing.

Next, move to your thighs. First, visualize the muscles very taught and tense, and then suddenly feel them release. Visualize the muscles completely relaxed.

Next let's move up to the buttocks. Visualize the gluteal muscles releasing all of their tension. If there is pressure on the nerve creating pain, visualize that muscle opening up so that the pain disseminates and the tension on the nerve goes away.

Now let's move up to our chest. If we hold most of our tension in our chest, when we close our eyes we can visualize the chest being constricted. As we take a slow, deep breath, visualize the rib cage expanding and all of those muscles completely relaxing. Then exhale and visualize the tension lifting off like steam out of the body. Take a deep inhale and, as you inhale, visualize inhaling a cool, very relaxing blue light. As the chest expands, the muscles relax. When you breathe out, visualize breathing out all of the dark, gray stress and toxins that are contained in your lungs and your chest.

Next, move to your neck and shoulders. If you have neck pain, you may visualize your neck with many, many knots, and muscle spasms. Go to each knot in the neck. Visualize the muscles in that knot unraveling one by one until the neck muscle becomes one smooth, lengthening muscle. Feel the tension lift and the pain disseminate. You feel lighter than air.

Finally, concentrate on your facial muscles. Visualize a smile on your face, the wrinkles of frowning smoothing out with a youthful look appearing. Take a deep breath in and visualize looking at yourself in the mirror, completely relaxed, lighter than air. Visualize a light, bright, white aura around your body. See yourself and bask in your deep relaxation.

Take a few more deep breaths and, when you are ready, open your eyes.

MEDITATION

The visualization exercise that you just completed can also be categorized as a type of meditation. **Meditation** can be done in five minutes, fifteen minutes, or an hour. It's simply setting aside quiet time to bring awareness and focus to your inner self.

Meditation can be done in stillness, but it can also be done in as part of an activity, such as yoga, running, free-form dancing, or any other activity that allows you to go into your inner self. It is designed to put you in connection with your higher consciousness.

MANTRAS

Mantras are commonly repeated words or phrases used to bring your awareness and focus to the present moment. Mantras are frequently used in meditation but do not have to be restricted to that. Mantras can be used at any time of the day during a stressful situation.

Two mantras that I like to use when in stressful situations are "And let that be okay" and "Acceptance is the key to my serenity today." Both help bring me back to the present moment rather than succumb to errant or erratic thoughts. They allow me to keep the focus on myself and to continue with the flow of life.

PRAYER

Prayer is the process of talking to your higher power or the God of your understanding. Some view prayer as a form of meditation. Some view it as both. Prayer can—and perhaps should—use the ideas we just reviewed. When you pray, you should relax. You may repeat a mantra. You may visualize. You may even make a declaration.

However and to whomever you pray, one thing is key: you must listen. Not with your ears, rather you listen internally. You will receive answers, or guidance, or resolve when you pray. Whether those come from the God of your belief or the Universe or your own (sub)consciousness doesn't matter. What matters is that you made a connection that will help you to progress.

SET YOUR OWN GOALS AND INTENTIONS

Now it is time for you to set your own goals and intentions. Remember that intentions and goals work together. Intentions are about the moment (they are realized in the present) and goals are about the future.

Remember the tools that you have available to help you get in touch with your true intentions and to help you set your goals: declarations, visualization, meditation, mantra, and prayer.

The most important thing is that it is a daily practice. Transformation does not happen overnight. Do not be hard on yourself if you don't get it right the first time or if you fall off the horse. Just jump right back on.

Don't quit!

Invest the time in yourself.

You are most certainly worth it.

4
LOVING YOURSELF
RESPONSIBLY
MEETING YOUR OWN NEEDS

PICTURE YOURSELF LYING ON A BEACH, WAVES crashing around you and you're feeling completely relaxed. You have had a hard month and you are taking a well-deserved weekend away. Your spouse agreed to take care of the children and you have left instructions only to be called in the case of an emergency. The phone rings. Your heart speeds up for fear of dreadful news. When you pick up the phone, it is your mother telling you that you need to call and talk to your sister right away because they had a big fight and she thinks that if you talked to her that maybe you could put some sense into her hard head. What do you do?

Often we get involved in things that are not our responsibility—and not even our business. We are so busy looking after others that we fail to see and tend to our own needs, resulting in undo stress and self-neglect.

RESPONSIBILITY AND OVER-RESPONSIBILITY

Taking care of yourself is an act of self-love and self-responsibility. The balance between these two is critical. When you are overly responsible, especially when it comes to other people's business, it usually is an indirect reflection of your own self-worth. Other examples of over-responsibility may be taking responsibility for things that are not yours, such as another person's feelings, actions, or uncontrollable events.

A client came into my office and told me that she thought that the man that she was about to marry may be an alcoholic. She was desperate to fix him, to get him into a program of recovery. Trying to fix her fiancé led her to become anxious, sleepless, nauseated, and, overall, a nervous wreck prior to the day that is supposed to be one of the happiest days for her. She was over-responsible—responsible for things that are not hers to be responsible for. In our sessions, we brought the focus back to her, dealing with the things that were in her control: her thoughts, her feelings, and her actions. Today, she is happily married with a baby on the way. She is able to be happy today because she rediscovered her worth and found the balance between being overly-responsible and self-responsible.

Having the right balance of self-love and self-responsibility will allow you to be able to take care of yourself and your well-being because you'll not only feel that you're worth it, but you'll give yourself permission *not* to take on other people's problems. You have enough love for yourself to know that you are not to blame for everything. On the flip-side, too little self-love can lead to under-responsibility or apathy. For example, if you feel like there's nothing you can do to make yourself pretty, you might neglect yourself by not going to the gym, not caring about what you eat, how you eat, or what you wear. Ultimately, this can compromise your health.

Is there such a thing as too much self-love? Extreme self-involvement can lead to selfishness and self-centered behaviors, which may negatively impact others, including family and friends. This is certainly not balance. However, there is a distinct difference between "loving yourself" and being classified as a "narcissist." A narcissistic person has a personality disorder in which the person is pathologically interested only in themselves and their well-being. A self-loving person, on the other hand, loves and respects others, just as he does himself.

Self-responsibility and self-love is the core of all other behaviors. It guides your decisions and the actions you take in life. In your notebook, write some personal examples of too much self-responsibility; not enough self-responsibility; too much self-love; and not enough self-love. Peruse those examples and write how they would affect the balance in your own life.

WHAT AFFECTS YOUR SENSE OF SELF-WORTH?

There are several things that can affect your self-esteem. One of them we visited in the last chapter: fear. There is an acronym that I learned for fear:

False **E**vidence **A**ppearing **R**eal

More often than not, the fears you hold are based on falsehoods that, for one reason or another, seem true and real to you. These fears may have been inculcated in you by family, friends, and colleagues. Here are some not-so-healthy messages that impart subtle fears and can ultimately affect your view of yourself.

"Don't speak unless you're spoken to." What is the underlying message here? The implied message is that if you speak your mind, there could be negative consequences. And nobody wants negative consequences, right?

"Playing sports is dangerous." The underlying message here is don't take risks. When I was in the seventh grade I played fast-pitch softball. During one game, the ball was hit into the outfield and it bounced and hit me square in the eye. My eye became swollen and I was bleeding. Being my mother's oldest and the first child to go through this, my mother completely freaked out. She made me quit the softball team and I didn't play sports until high school. I wanted to play volleyball in the ninth grade and begged my mom to let me play. Finally, she let me join the volleyball team. It was a great experience to be able to take that risk because I became quite an avid volleyball player. Had she not allowed me to join that volleyball team, it may have embedded further the message that it was too risky and that taking any kind of risk was not safe and not in my best interest, ever.[1]

"If you want anything done right, you have to do it yourself." Underlying message: Don't trust anyone. Of

[1] On a side note about my mother, she is a risk taker and she is a living example that being fearless and taking risks can lead to incredible success. So whereas I learned an early message that taking risk can be dangerous, i.e. the softball in the eye, I also learned the message from her that when you do take a risk and be a trailblazer, that you can have insurmountable success and fulfillment in life.

course, knowing who and who not to trust is a great skill to have and it is very important to be able to take care of yourself. But not trusting *anyone* can ultimately lead to over-responsibility, isolation, and, eventually, to you feeling overwhelmed and alone. I am definitely a living testament to being overwhelmed because I was given the message early on in life that I had to do things that I wanted done correctly. Later in my life I learned that it is okay to trust safe people and ask for help. Knowing who is safe and who is not safe is the key to knowing who to trust.[2]

We also receive many false messages from our social environment. The nay-sayers out there who are "no-no-ing" you to death are projecting their own fears onto you. This usually comes in the form of a friend or a colleague discouraging you from trying something new because of their bad experience or an experience that they heard from someone else. They may make discouraging statements like "It's too hard to start your own business," "My friend was a vegetarian and still died from cancer," "This one doctor didn't even know what the diagnosis was," or "Be careful about going to those chiropractors, they can break your neck." All of these statements are based on incomplete or false information, but they ingrain a fear that is subconscious and substantial, influencing you and sometimes preventing you from taking action.[3]

---

2 That will come in a later chapter in this book.
3 I know personally, if I had listened to the fears ingrained by my colleagues, I would not be a successful wellness coach and consultant, appearing on television programs to give expert advice – and I certainly wouldn't be writing this book. In short, I could not make a difference in the lives of others in the way that I do today if I listened to every fear-based comment made by those around me.

Overcoming these fears comes in two main processes. The first is recognizing that you are worthy and that you are a child of God (or whatever Higher Power you believe in); that you are a person of worth.

The second is retraining your brain and resetting that internal dialogue that you have with yourself, something that we will talk more about later in this book.

When you live in fear you miss out on being your authentic self. The cost is happiness, self esteem, self-expression, and, ultimately, your well-being. In short, you miss out on life. Recognizing that fear is **F**alse **E**vidence **A**ppearing **R**eal is of paramount importance. Will fears go away? No! However, by recognizing fear for what it is, it will have less of a grip over you and your choices. More on that later.

Another aspect of fear that affects our view of self is **self-doubt**. Self-doubt relates to both fear and potentially faulty belief systems. But why do we doubt our abilities?

The answer will be different for each individual, but for some, the choice not to believe in one's abilities is rooted in **fear of success**. When you choose to accept the responsibility of being worthy, you have to accept the responsibility of your ability to overcome your obstacles. Then, you actually have to take action. For some, the action may seem overwhelming, especially when you don't know where to start. These are cases when having a support structure that helps you, such as a wellness coach, can be very valuable in the process of making life more manageable. When I work with patients and clients, I help them not only to see the root of their faulty belief systems, but also to identify what it is that they really want. Together, we create small steps that make moving through and around potential blocks much less daunting and much more doable. Usually, the client becomes so efficient, that within a few weeks, they are setting their own action steps. And further down the road, they are achieving their goals! In short, get help when you think you need it. Remember that a significant part of self-love is to allow yourself to ask for help. There's no shame in that—only the chance for greater success.

There are also external factors and blocks that sometimes delay you from getting to where you want to go, such as time and money. Ultimately, though, it is your own self-placed barriers that hold you back from being your true authentic self and that ultimately affects your own sense of self-worth and self-responsibility. Often, we use external factors or influences as excuses for why we are not able to complete a task. There may have been a time where you were victimized in your life. There may have been a time when this victimization lowered your self-esteem or caused you to feel overly responsible for things not yours. As adults, we all have choices—and we can either *choose* to continue being victims or we can choose to become participants in our own lives.

Building self-love and self-esteem can be a process or it can be a simple choice. It may seem trite, but loving yourself starts with the simple acts of love and authenticity.

SELF-LOVE BUILDING EXERCISES
Proclaim your love for yourself. When you awaken in the morning, look yourself in the mirror and say to

yourself, "I love you!" It may sound corny, but do it any-way. As science has shown, the more we say something, the more that we believe it. As you do the action, the be-lief will come.

Perform estimable acts. An estimable act may be as simple as acting on someone else's behalf or even acting on your own behalf.

Set and respect your own boundaries. That may seem counter-intuitive, but it is the very act of setting boundar-ies that gives you the room to then take the extra steps for your own self-care. In fact, setting boundaries, which we will explore later in this book, is in itself an act of self-care.

LOVE AND RESPECT THYSELF

Promoting self-love by loving yourself will turn into the fuel of self-responsibility because your emotional tank will be full. If your emotional tank is empty, what do you have to give to others?

Practicing self-love and balancing it with self-respon-sibility is a daily application. However, it is the core and the foundation for all of the other steps that we're going to encounter in this book. And when you do daily apply the principles of self-love and self-responsibility, you'll begin to feel the shift in yourself and you'll be motivated to take the next step.

PART II

FLOOR PLAN

The way you think, the way you behave, the way you eat, can influence your life by 30 to 50 years.

—Dr. Deepak Chopra

5
BE MINDFUL, BE STILL
THE BREATH OF LIFE

CAN YOU PICTURE YOURSELF SITTING CROSS-legged in the middle of the floor of one of the rooms of your home, eyes closed, hands on knees in the typical yoga position breathing and chanting, "Ohm"? Neither can most people.

Unfortunately, that's how most people envision meditating. They think it's something gurus or swamis do that involves strange poses and even stranger chants. While that's somewhat true for some styles of meditation, the good news is that if this style of meditation is not for you, then you are *not* out of luck!

Simply put, meditation is a state of constant awareness and focus on the present moment. It can come in many forms: breathing, moving, sensing, feeling, eating, and creating. At its heart, meditation is a sort of biofeedback to the brain—you give the command and the brain follows.

This chapter has techniques that you can use to achieve a state of awareness so that you can better control yourself, your life, and your health. It all begins with something we do everyday without even thinking about it: breathing.

THE HEALING POWER OF MEDITATION

I was on vacation in Rhode Island. It was extremely hot and sunny and, due to activities and excursions, I hadn't slept much. That was bad: two triggers for a migraine were triggered. What was worse: I had none of my migraine medication with me.

A migraine is not just a "bad headache." It's an entire syndrome of fatigue, tensions, light sensitivity, even nausea and dizziness. It can be a very painful and debilitating ailment. For migraine sufferers, having a migraine and not having medication can be very scary.

I could feel the tension in my neck building and my head was starting to throb. When the light sensitivity began, I knew I was in trouble, as that is one of the classic symptoms of the onset of a migraine. Even though I didn't have my medication, I did have my mp3 player, which contained numerous guided meditations, one specifically for headaches and pain. With no other option, I decided to find a quiet place to sit and try this meditation.

For forty minutes I meditated. I focused on my breathing. I relaxed myself to release my tension. I visualized pain leaving my head, neck, and shoulders.

When I was finished, I was free of any pain. I was able to prevent a migraine by breathing, relaxing, and visualizing.

I relate this story to you to make a point: many people believe that meditation is just for relaxation or stress relief or that it's even some sort of "woo." The fact is that it is based in science. Meditation is a biofeedback system that can control how the brain releases substances like neurotransmitters and hormones to help you to balance and achieve your desired state of mind.

As a doctor, I am a firm believer in meditation as a source of reducing pain and stress. I use meditation techniques with my clients for various issues including anxiety, insomnia, pain, negative thinking, and for opening and centering during the coaching process. Often my patients come back to me reporting great progress with as little as 5-10 minutes of breathing exercise.[1]

PROPER BREATHING

Imagine yourself reducing stress and feeling centered and more productive. If you suffer from headaches or migraines, imagine yourself pain-free. If you suffer from insomnia, imagine getting a good night's rest. You can attain all of that—and more—with simple breathing techniques.

The deep breath is emotionally stabilizing and it helps in acutely stressful situations. It does this by activating the parasympathetic nervous system—the division of the nervous system responsible for regulating your internal organs and glands—so that you can make effective decisions during adrenaline producing situations.

As we talk about mindfulness, which is really being in the present moment, we're integrating that with meditation in its different forms. But the core of meditation is the breath.

1 Having had the pain of migraines for years, I can tell you that I have no reservation about taking medication to alleviate debilitating pain. Or, for that matter, taking the proper medication for any ailment I may have. Meditation can be a very powerful tool in your health and wellness toolbox. Just as you wouldn't use a hammer to screw a screw, so you shouldn't shun proper medication as prescribed by a doctor for your ailments.

Breathing is something that is involuntary and, therefore, we often take it for granted. But breathing fully and slowly has been shown to affect many processes in the body and the mind. Breathing as a feedback has been scientifically proven to:

△ Lower blood pressure

△ Stop panic attacks

△ Promote deep restful sleep

△ Center the mind

△ Stop negative or obsessive thoughts

△ Help with mental focus and clarity

△ Increase oxygen delivery to muscles and organs

△ Increases exercise performance

Ultimately, when you allow yourself to fully and properly breathe, you will achieve an overall relaxing experience. So, let's look at how breathing plays an important role in the other dimensions of wellness.

When you take a deep breath, how do you feel? If you're in a stressful situation when you take a deep breath, how do you communicate? When you allow yourself to breathe deeply, how is your thought process? When you're breathing properly, how are you eating? Are you stuffing your face or are you allowing yourself to enjoy your food?

You can see that just simple mindfulness with the breath can affect all the different areas in the wellness energy system. To that aim, here is a quick coherence meditation that will help you center yourself and get you breathing properly in as little as five minutes. Read the meditation first, then try it.

COHERENCE MEDITATION

Take a comfortable position, either seated or lying down. Begin to take slow, deep breaths—in and out, in and out. As you're taking deep breaths, bring your focus to the center of your chest, which we will call your heart center. Continue to breathe deeply, in and out. As you're breathing, with your heart center, begin to focus on breathing into your heart and out of your heart. Imagine, as you breathe in, the air goes into your heart and fills your chest. When you breathe out, it's coming out of your chest. You can imagine bringing a clear, bright, sparkly light into your chest as you breathe in and breathe out the gray, dark stress. Continue focusing on your heart and breathing. Now, as you're continuing this heart breathing, bring into focus something that you feel grateful for or something that makes you feel good. Continue to breathe. Notice the feeling in your body as you focus on what you're grateful for and hold that space as you breathe it into your heart. As you breathe in, holding this space of gratitude and good feeling, notice a shift in how your body feels. When you are ready, open your eyes and come back to the present.

How do you feel? This is a simple, four to five minute meditation that you can do any time of the day. As you do this meditation on a daily basis, you will begin to notice changes in your own body and in your own mindset.

ANOTHER FORM OF MINDFULNESS

Now let's talk about another form of mindfulness. This comes through accessing our five senses—taste, touch, smell, sight, and hearing. People often get confused whenever I talk about the senses affecting the other dimensions, so I frame it as how the other dimensions may affect our senses and how the stressors in our life may affect our senses.

Let's do a quick mini-inventory and break down the senses into their five elements.

What does stress do to the senses?

What does stress do to your taste?

What does stress do to your sense of touch?

What does your stress do to your sense of smell?

When you are stressed out, how is your sight, or your seeing dimension?

When you are stressed out, how is your hearing, or more importantly, how is your filter of hearing?

Gaining mindfulness—or coming back to the present—by accessing our senses is a great way to get back into your body and to see and experience the world for how beautiful and vivid it really is. Here's another mindfulness exercise that you can do accessing the senses through a walk or even a drive. I'll use the example of walking, but if you're in the car, then you can do this, taking care to pay attention to your surroundings so that you don't have an accident. Read the meditation, then try it on your own.

SENSORY WALK

Let's go for a 25-minute walk. I can be anywhere: in a

park, along a path you know, down the street. Try to make it as free of other people as possible. In this examples here, I'm taking us on a walk on a path. Ready? Let's go.

For the first five minutes, you're only to notice what you *see*. As you're walking, notice the bright colors around you, notice the details of the flowers, the ground, the rocks. Concentrate on all of the colors.

After the first five minutes, you're only to notice what you *hear*. Of course you'll be watching where you're going so as not to have an accident, but consciously activate your sense of hearing. Do you hear birds chirping? Do you hear crickets? Do you hear cars passing by? Listen to the wind, or even listen to the silence.

For next five-minute span, you're to notice what you *smell*. If you're walking outside in the morning, are you smelling the dew in the air? Is there an impending rainfall and you can smell the moisture? You might smell the flowers or the trees or freshly cut grass.

In the next five minutes, you're to activate your sense of *touch*. Notice the breeze on your skin as you're walking. Notice the feel of your clothing brushing against your skin; your hair dropping by your shoulders or back; the temperature of your skin. Do you feel warm and comfortable? Do you feel chilly? Really activate that sense of touch. It brings you right to the present.

Finally, you're to activate your sense of *taste*. If you're chewing gum, you might taste the minty flavor. You might taste the moisture in the air or the sweetness of the flowers that you just smelled. Or maybe you're walking by someone's house and they're cooking and you taste the scent of whatever is being cooked.

Here you've had a 25-minute sensory walk. It should have brought you into the present moment, allowing you to really experience your body and interact with the world on a very physical level. If you do this a couple of times a week, you will notice that you'll naturally begin to pay attention more to what you see and to what you hear and the beauty of your surroundings. You're integrating this into your system, and it will help relax you, bringing you to a more serene place.

YOUR CREATIVE SELF

Another way to center your mind is to utilize **your creative self.** That is the part of you that yearns to create, whether that creativity is explored through writing, singing, playing a musical instrument, painting, drawing, or whatever else you can imagine.

I use poetry to access my creative self. I've been writing since I was twelve years old and I can honestly say that writing poetry has saved my life. In 2004, I began performing spoken word, and that took me to a whole other level of creativity and mindfulness. Being on stage and sharing my innermost feelings and writings with others compelled me to find a sense of comfort with myself. This also relates to self-love: I loved myself enough to know that my experiences made me the strong and compassionate person that I am today. That allowed—and continues to allow—me to be able to share some of my poetry with the world. When I used to host an open mic night, I would have to be in the present moment to be able to engage and interact with the audience from moment to moment, improvising and making people laugh. Being able to do this improved my public speaking skills, making me a more dynamic and spontaneous presenter. Yes, this type of mindfulness can flow into other areas of your life.

Now, I'm not suggesting that you go and host an open mic night or get in front of a large audience if you don't want to. What I am saying is that infusing creativity into your daily life can help you to balance yourself both emotionally and spiritually. It promotes your overall wellness by making you notice and be present in yourself at each moment—with your feelings, actions, and connections with others.

I use this in my practice by helping my clients remember what they love to do and ask them to infuse their own creativity as a source of relaxation and mindfulness. Some use cooking, some use photography, and some use writing poetry and short stories as a way to be present.

What are your sources of creativity? Do you like performing or acting or singing? Are you involved with an art such as painting, sculpting, textiling, crocheting, knitting, or sewing? Maybe you like pottery or jewelry making? What are other sources of creativity that you might not have even considered before?

I've heard many people say, "Well I don't have a creative bone in my body." But everyone—everyone!—has a creative side. It's just a matter of finding your inspiration. What are your sources of inspiration? Are there people in your life—your family, friends, coworkers—who provide you with inspiration? If you're a person who sees clients or patients, do they inspire you? Are there places that you go frequently or imagine that give you vision?[2] For some there are certain situations that may be a catalyst for writing or speaking. There may be internal emotional sources of inspiration. If you're going through a traumatic situation or even a joyful situation, this may be a muse for you. There may be spiritual sources, like music. Whatever the source, it is important to acknowledge your creative self and to know that there are consequences for not doing so.

YOUR WELLNESS AND YOUR CREATIVE SELF

Let's look at some consequences by checking against our other areas of well-being.

When I am not in my creative self, my self-responsibility and self-love are _____.

When I am not in my creative self, my breathing is _____.

When I am not in my creative self, my senses are _____.

When I am not in my creative self, my eating is _____.

When I am not in my creative self, my feeling is _____.

When I am not in my creative self, my movement is

_____.

---

2 I personally love nature. There is a park around the corner from where I live that has a stream. It's so inspirational for me to be able to just sit by the running water and listen to all the sounds around it. It helps me to concentrate and focus and access my inner self.

When I am not in my creative self, my communicating is _____.

When I am not in my creative self, my thinking is _____.

When I am not in my creative self, my working and playing balance is _____.

When I am not in my creative self, my intimate or close relationships are _____.

When I am not in my creative self, my ability to find meaning in life is _____.

When I am not in my creative self, my connection with my higher source is _____.

Now we ask the question, what are the things that help us to access our creativity? Before we answer that question, let's do one more mindfulness exercise. Let's look at how each dimension affects your creativity.

How does your self-love and self-responsibility help you to access your creativity?

How does your breathing, your eating, and your sensing dimensions help you to access that creativity?

How does your feelings help you access your creativity?

How does your movements help you access your creativity?

How do your communication styles help you access your creativity?

How do your thoughts help you to access your creativity?

How does your work or how does your play help you to access your creativity?

How do your close relationships and your connection with others help you to access your creativity?

How does what life means to you help you to access that creativity?

How does your connection with your higher source help you to access that creativity?

Again, as you complete this exercise reflect on the ways that these different dimensions either help or hinder your access to that creativity, and how when you're not in your creative self each of these dimensions is affected.

GETTING INTO YOUR CREATIVE SELF

Now let's talk about some ways that you can get into your creative self. Some people refer to this as "getting into the zone," where the "zone" is that mental place where you are completely focused and fixated on the present moment.

Still your mind. We talked about meditation earlier. We talked about proper breathing and we took a sensory walk. These are ways to relax yourself so that you are more open to receiving inspiration. Like I wrote earlier, meditation comes in different forms; it may be yoga, it may be running or some other type of exercise, dancing, or writing. Any way that you find focus into your mind, any activity that you can do to still your mind, will create an openness for you to be able to receive inspiration.

Affirmations. We talked about how to create affirmations earlier in this book. The concept of affirming yourself in various ways is one that will resurface in all areas of your life. Say this affirmation aloud: *I am the source of creativity and expression.* Notice how you feel. Create an affirmation of your own so that your mind begins to open your creative soul.

Intuition. Later on in this book, we will discuss creating flow through intuition in much more detail. However, a fun exercise to try now is to choose a day and let everything you do be guided by your intuitive self. This will allow you to experience what it's like to do things from your higher self rather than from society's view of what you should be doing all day every day.

Ask Your Higher Source. If you believe in God or a higher power, then a wonderful way of receiving inspiration is simply to ask your higher source. Spiritual practices such as prayer can help you to become more open to that inspiration that will help you to access your creative self.

Journaling. Writing about your day, your feelings, and your experiences is a great way to bring out your creative side. There's an exercise that I like to do called *free writing*. Pick a topic—a person, a situation, an event—and begin to write whatever comes to your mind about it. Don't put a time limit on yourself; just write until the pen runs dry (or your hand gets cramped). It may not make sense at the time, but if you go back and read what you wrote you may pull some very creative and inspiring tidbits that you may not have thought that you felt.

A similar exercise is to set a timer for five minutes and then write whatever comes to your mind about whatever topic. The topic doesn't matter. It doesn't have to make sense. Just write. This is sort of an emotional purging of sorts. It's very helpful to do this before you go to bed at night. It actually helps you to sleep better. You can read your entry a couple of days later; you may find that it is very insightful in accessing your inner emotional self as well as accessing your inner creativity.

Sensory walk. As we saw earlier, this accesses your observing self. As you walk around and you're accessing what you're seeing and what you're hearing, you can then come back and write or paint or sculpt or whatever other type of activity that you like to do from that inspiration.

Play. Even as we grow older, we still need some play in our lives. You can involve your family, your children, your spouse, and your friends. Play time is great to bring out the creativity in others because we're not so caught up in thinking about what we have to do as we become emotionally free when we play and we have the opportunity to just experience our natural selves.

Let's end this section with a few quick *anywhere meditations*. These are meditations that, as the name implies, you can do anywhere at just about any time. They're quick "snacks" when you don't have the opportunity for a complete "meal."

Close your eyes. Just about no matter where you are,

you can always close your eyes.[3] It takes you away from the in-the-moment chaos and allows you some space from the situation.

Say a prayer. You don't have to believe in God to say a prayer. A prayer can be sort of like a mantra. Make it short and sweet and one that you know well. I personally like "The Serenity Prayer" and I've found that it has worked well with many of my clients and patients.

> God, grant me the serenity to accept the things I
> cannot change, the courage to change the things
> that I can, and the wisdom to know the difference.

Saying a simple mantra or prayer such as this also helps to take you out of the current situation and into yourself, allowing you space and the opportunity to center yourself.

Take five. If you're having a very stressful day and you found yourself in the middle of chaos, walk away for five minutes. Usually, five minutes is just enough time to recenter yourself and to refill your tank.

Ten breaths and a smile. Close your eyes, take ten slow and deep breaths, and, at the end of the tenth breath, just smile. Even if you're not feeling like it, the smile at the end of the tenth breath will give you a good feeling and help you to move on through your day.

PUTTING IT ALL TOGETHER

Proper breathing is the cornerstone of wellness.

---

3 Of course you don't want to close your eyes if you're driving or operating heavy machinery. You can close your eyes, however, if you're in your car at a red light. Just remember to open your eyes before the light turns green so you don't make the drivers behind you horn-happy!

Meditation and mindfulness based on proper breathing can heal and promote good health because it acts on many aspects of our nervous system.

As we practice meditative techniques, we also tap into our creativity.

Our creativity then becomes a part of our meditative practice.

As you can see, one thing builds upon the other. Each influences and affects the other. Just like the parts of a house (or any other building) influence each other. If you have a weak foundation, your house will topple. If you're floors are unsupported, you will fall through.

Follow *The Wellness Blueprint* as it's presented here. I made these exercises and activities easy and accessible so that any person in any circumstances can practice them. The end result—as each exercise builds upon other exercises and as each exercise influences other exercises—is you reclaiming your health and wellness.

With that in mind, it might be time for a snack. So, we'll talk about eating next.

6
You Are What (and How) You Eat
Garbage In, Garbage Out

THE MOST COMMON THING WE HEAR FROM OUR doctors about maintaining our health is what? Diet and exercise! It seems so simple: eat right and stay active. Unfortunately, simple doesn't always mean easy. If it were easy, then we'd already be doing it and you wouldn't be reading this book. Which is why I want to focus this chapter on how we can make what seems difficult manageable.

ENJOYABLE EATING

Imagine yourself at ten years old. Did you enjoy eating? Did you enjoy family dinners with conversation or lunch hour with your friends at school? Eating is supposed to be enjoyable and enjoyable eating can be nutritious as well as time efficient.

Most people understand what is and isn't nutritious and what constitutes a balanced diet. However, sometimes the choices we make don't reflect that knowledge. Why is it that we continue to make unhealthy choices when we know the consequences of our behavior? This is a question that I have asked patients over and over again. The most common answer is the overwhelming feeling that comes with having to give up all of the things that they love. Some people get overwhelmed at the thought of starting a new behavior, such as going through their kitchen and throwing out the bad food and starting from scratch. Others may know what foods are healthy, but they cannot translate that to cooking or creating meals. We will discuss issues like these, but first, let's look at how the actual process of eating affects us and how we can be mindful about it.

Where do you eat? Do you sit at a dinner table with family? Do you eat in the car? Where we eat is just as important as what or how we eat. We're all guilty of "grabbing a quick bite" or snacking at our desk. And those are acceptable from time to time. Your aim, though, should be to be mindful of your eating—and where you eat aids you in that.

What do you do while you eat? Do you talk on the phone? Work on your computer? Multi-task in some other way? Again, mindfulness is your aim. When you allow distractions while you eat, you detract from any attempts you may try at mindfulness. That can lead to other problems.

How about chewing? Do you chew your food properly? Or do you just "inhale" it due to lack of time? How do you think not chewing your food affects your digestion? I'll tell you how. When you don't chew your food properly, it puts a strain on your stomach and intestines because those organs then have to do the job that your teeth should have done.

How about what you do after you eat? If you lay down soon after you eat, you block the natural pathway of food digestion. Remember to remain upright for at least an hour to two hours after your meal. This allows gravity to assist in the downward movement of the food into the intestines.

Putting all of these ideas together, here is a mindfulness eating meditation that you can practice. Like the other meditations we've done so far, it's easy.

Choose one meal during your day where you can sit down in a quiet place. Sit at a table in a comfortable chair where you're upright. You can either sit in silence or you can play your favorite relaxing music in the background. Eat your meal relatively slowly, chewing each bite at least 25 to 50 times. You may close your eyes and savor the different flavors and the different textures. Experience the enjoyment of the taste of the food. When you feel satisfied, not full, stop eating.

When you eat just one meal a day in this fashion, you will feel lighter and less bloated and find that your food digests much better. Additionally, when you chew your food properly and eat a little bit more slowly, you will tend to eat fewer calories and decrease digestion problems such as heartburn or gastric reflux.

WHAT YOU EAT

What do you think are the most common excuses that people make for poor eating? The most common excuses that I hear are "I don't have time to cook" and "I'm too tired to cook when I get home" and "I don't have any help." What other excuses can you think of? These excuses (and yours) may be valid; what we want to do, though, is to create a more manageable situation and learn how healthy cooking and eating can be time efficient and easier than you might think.

Let's first talk about the basics of healthy eating.

Portion control. Monitoring the portions of food you serve yourself is very important in maintaining your weight. It's easy to do, too. Take a round, regular-sized plate and divide it into four sections:

Δ   ¼ of the plate is for starches or carbohydrates;

Δ   ¼ of the plate for meat or protein,

Δ   ½ of the plate is for vegetables.

This is the easy way to measure so that you get your four to six servings of vegetables a day and you don't over-do it on the proteins and the carbohydrates.

Ideally, we should be taking five to six small meals a day. Broken down, that is three "traditional" meals (breakfast, lunch, and dinner) and two small snacks in between.

Servings. How many serving of fruits and vegetables to you eat per day? The proper amount of servings for vegetables is four to six servings a day. That is approximately one to two vegetables per meal or snack. Fruit? Ideally, most people should get three to four servings of fruit a day, which is simple when you use fruit as a snack.[1] Protein requirements are between 25 to 30 grams per a day.

---

1   This amount will vary for diabetics. If you are diabetic, check with your physician.

Keep in mind that there are more sources of protein than just meat, such as beans, legumes, soy-based meat substitutes like tofu, or gluten-based substitutes like seitan. As for fiber, the average person needs 25 to 35 grams of fiber in their diet each day. Fiber is very important because not only does it lower cholesterol, it also lowers blood pressure, lowers the risk of colon cancers, and helps you to lose weight by keeping things moving through the intestinal system.

This is a very basic nutritional overview. Please see the back of this book for more references. Before we move to meal planning, here is a list of supplements that are essential for any household.

Potent Multivitamin. Even if you are getting the proper amount of servings of fruits, vegetables, protein, and fiber, you should still take a daily multivitamin. The soil that foods are grown in today are not as nutrient rich as they used to be and vitamin and mineral deficiencies are much more prevalent today. The best vitamins to get are liquid because they are more bioavailable and more easily absorbed. I personally like the Buried Treasure VM-100 Complete, but there are many potent liquid vitamins that are of quality out there.

Superfood Greens. Super green supplements such as wheat grass, barley grass, spirulina, or chlorella are blood building and are great sources of antioxidants. They also lower blood pressure, cholesterol, increase the immune response, and are anti-inflammatory in nature. I particularly like Green Vibrance by Vibrant Health.

Omega Supplement. Omega supplements are anti-inflammatory in nature and great for mood stability and brain development. Most people take fish oils, of which there are many combinations: Omega 3, Omega 3-6-9, and Flaxseed combinations. If you are a vegetarian, there is a supplement called EFA-Health from the Sun, that combines flaxseed with evening primrose and borage seed oil. Otherwise, I recommend Krill Oil 1000mg Daily.[2] Krill Oil has been shown in studies to reduce inflammation in arthritis and lower LDL (Low-density lipoprotein, also known as the "bad cholesterol") and triglycerides (fat in the blood) more so then traditional fish oils.

Probiotics and Prebiotics. With all of the antibiotics that doctors prescribe (not to mention the antibiotics in the meats that people eat), probiotics are necessary to prevent "leaky gut syndrome"[3] from overgrowth of yeast or bad bacteria in our bodies. Probiotics are healthy bacteria that we ingest to help our digestion. Prebiotics are fibers that nourishes the healthy bacteria already in our digestive tract. There are many combinations of probiotics, but the product that I mentioned earlier, Green Vibrance, has plenty of prebiotics and probiotics.

Co-enzyme Q 10. For those who have a family history or a personal history of hypertension, diabetes, or heart disease of any kind, 100mg of Co-enzyme Q-10, preferably with Alpha Lipoic Acid (ALA) is a very important addition to your supplement regimen to protect your

---

2 Unless you are allergic to shellfish.
3 While not a medical diagnosis, "leaky gut syndrome" refers to a bevy of symptoms including bloating, cramps, flatulence, aches, and pains.

heart and blood vessels. It has been shown to reduce the risk of heart disease and complications.

Vitamin D. For women, calcium and Vitamin D are very important to protect the bones and prevent osteoporosis. However, studies are now showing that deficiency in Vitamin D may have a role in increased risk for heart disease. Since sun exposure is the main way that our skin activates Vitamin D production, we are finding more and more Vitamin D deficiency today due to the fact that we spend most of our days indoors. It is essential to get it checked at your regular doctor visits and, if low, supplement with 1000mg daily until your levels are normal.

MEAL PLANNING

Now that you know how to eat and what to eat, let's get to making those great meals. A major way to make healthy eating more manageable and, therefore, more enjoyable, is to plan your meals.

I know! I can hear the groans all the way over here. In the past, the woman would stay home and plan and prepare meals while the man would go to work. Fortunately, times have changed and we are no longer bound to those strict gender roles. But, like "blood is the price of freedom," meal planning is the price of equality and opportunity, as well as health and wellness. If you find this difficult, then go back a few chapters and review your priorities. Remember what you want to accomplish and how much you want to reclaim your health and wellness.

With all that said, plan your meals for the week. I know that may seem hard, especially if you have a family and career that you have to think about. Help yourself make it easier: have a quick family meeting to discuss what everyone would like for meals during the week. (Of course, if you are single, then you'd make a meal plan for yourself.) What this family meeting does is gets the whole family participating in the healthy eating idea. Remember, if you're the parent, then you are the role model to your children; if you're married, then you're a significant influence on your spouse. Making this process as light and enjoyable as possible will give your family a positive association with being healthy. Having a "family meeting" doesn't mean you have to become a made-to-order chef. All it's meant to accomplish it to give you some ideas of what you will need when you are making your list to go shopping.

Meal planning includes breakfast, lunch, snacks, and dinner. Keep that in mind when you are making your shopping list. For example, lunch may be a leftover and it also may be packed the night before for efficiency. Snacks may be prepared beforehand so all you need to do is grab and go, such as sliced fruit cups or bags of granola.

Next, you will prepare your shopping list—and, therefore, do your shopping—according to the meal plan. Not only will you shopping take less time, it will also be more economical. Plan to grocery shop weekly as this will prevent you from over-buying (which saves money and lessens waste) and will encourage you to buy fresh rather than packaged and preserved.

While we're on the topic of shopping, here are a few grocery store tips. First, he best place to shop is the farmer's market because they have the freshest produce. They also tend to have more organic dairy and meats and the meats tend to be fresher and not cleaned with the bleaches that the grocery stores tend to have. However, I understand that not everybody has access to a farmer's market or some may only have access seasonally (such as during the summer). Worry not; you can stay healthy and still shop at your local grocery store.

When you go to the grocery store, typically, produce, meats, frozen foods, and dairy are on the perimeter. Shopping the perimeter of the grocery store first is the best strategy to avoid picking up junk foods and unhealthy, prepackaged, processed foods. In fact, you primarily want to stick to the perimeter of the grocery store because once you start getting into the middle, you run into snacks, sodas, pasta, and all the things you don't need that can be tempting.

In the store, make it a habit to reading labels. Look for the amount of fiber, carbohydrates, sugar, sodium, protein and the fat. You will be surprised what happens to the desire to buy junk when you begin reading the labels.

Never go shopping on an empty stomach. When you're hungry, you're more likely to impulse shop and buy things that you absolutely know you wouldn't buy if your stomach were full. Have a full meal or a solid snack before you go grocery shopping. It will keep your mind clear and focused on your shopping list.

If you can, get an accountability partner. This can be of great help if you tend to have a low resistance for the junk foods once they are in front of you. Text or call them if you're getting overly tempted by the junk foods. It's amazing what a little support from a friend can do for your will power.

Finally, always take a shopping list and stick to it. Buy only what's on the list. And forgo any impulse buys.

QUICK AND EASY FOOD PREPARATION

Casseroling. This is one of my personal favorites. Casseroling keeps all of the parts of your meal (vegetables, starches, protein) in one dish. It's easy to pack and take with you for lunch the next day. A couple of classics that I like are broccoli, chicken and rice casserole and tuna casserole. They're very easy to make. Use whole grain pasta and brown rice for better nutritional value.

Steaming. Steaming is very quick and easy method of preparation that can provide a well-balanced meal. Any vegetable can be steamed. Even fish can be seasoned and steamed. The typical preparation time for steaming vegetables is about five minutes. Steaming keeps vegetables crisp and keeps them from being overcooked; it also allows them to retain their nutritional value. Add a little sea salt and pepper on top, even sprinkle a little Parmesan cheese or lemon pepper.

Fish (or other seafood) might take a little bit longer because it's a protein, but it still steams fairly quickly. Marinade the fish in advance or sprinkle some of your favorite herbs on top.

If you're new to steaming, you might want to go about purchasing a steaming kit which basically consists of a large pot with a steam basket. This makes steaming so much easier. I don't recommend using a microwave oven to steam your food as microwaving alters the nutrients of the food.

Stir frying. Stir frying vegetables alone or with a protein (chicken, shrimp, tofu) takes no more than 15-20 minutes. All you need is a wok—either a fancy electric wok or traditional stove top wok. Add just a bit of olive oil to cover the bottom of the wok, then add your chopped vegetables (either frozen previously or you can use them fresh), and sauté them until they're lightly cooked. If you're adding a protein, pan sear it while you're chopping your vegetables. Shrimp cooks very quickly so you only need cook it for about five to ten minutes before you add it to your stir fry.

Pan searing. Another quick and easy prep method. It's great for a protein like salmon or chicken breast. That along with a steamed vegetable and some brown rice or quinoa or cous cous is an excellent, healthy, and tasty meal.

Sautéing. I primarily use sautéing with scallops, shrimp, and vegetables. You can also sauté rice after it's cooked and even pasta.

Pressure Cooking. Pressure cooking is a little bit different because it allows you to cook things that normally would take longer, like black beans or red beans or even your brown or wild grain rices, in a very short amount of time. For example, typically black beans take about an hour to cook to a proper consistency; with a pressure cooker, you can make them and rice in about 30 minutes. You can find a good pressure cooker at just about any decent retailer. I can assure you that it is definitely worth the purchase because it opens up so much more of a variety of foods that you can cook in under a half-hour that you otherwise might have wanted to avoid.

HEALTHY AND DELICIOUS

Herbs and spices are wonderful ways to "punch up" your food. You can use them on their own by putting them on your food. A dash of paprika or a touch of garlic can make just about any protein magical.

Marinades are another thing to keep in mind. By combining a few herbs and spices with some olive oil or other base liquid transforms a simple protein into a complex treat for the tongue. Marinades can even be effective tenderizers for proteins that tend to get "tough" when prepared.

Orange and pineapple juice in apple cider or balsamic vinaigrette and olive oil create a wonderful marinade or a salad dressing. If you like a Caribbean flavor, go with jerk seasoning or even curry. Curry, tumeric, coriander and cumin also make great Indian style dishes. Other traditional herbs to include in your cooking are thyme, basil, marjoram, and dill weed. You can combine thyme, basil, marjoram, sea salt, and a red or white wine vinegar or a cooking wine to create a wonderful marinade. Take dill weed, thyme, and white wine vinegar, add an organic mushroom soup, and you have a great chicken, beef, or scallop sauce. Look online for more ideas. You won't have any trouble finding simple yet inventive recipes.

Eating Out Or On the Go

What about making healthy choices when you can't cook or when you just don't like to cook? All of the "rules" we discussed in this chapter still apply: when you feel satisfied, then stop eating; watch your portion size; vegetables should comprise the greater share of the meal. Simple.

Here are some restaurant tips and ideas that you should follow. You may already know, some of them. It's good to be reminded, though.

△   Order the steamed vegetables on the side instead of the starch.

△   Get butter, salad dressings, or sauces on the side.

△   Split your meal with whomever you're eating.

△   Split your meal with yourself. Ask for a to-go box as soon as the food comes out. Place half of that food into the box.

△   Make a meal of an appetizer. (With the portions sizes in some restaurants these days, this is making more and more sense. Plus, it often saves a lot of money.)

△   If you must stop at a fast food restaurant, consider the soup and salad option.

△   Dip your salad bites into the dressing instead of pouring it over the salad. That way you can get the full taste of the dressing on each bite without slathering the whole salad and destroying the nutritional value of the salad in the first place.

△   Try a deli or a sandwich place instead of your traditional fast food restaurant.

Δ Order wraps.

Δ Avoid fried anything.

Δ Go for the salad and light dressing.

Δ Go light on cheesy appetizers and entrées.

Δ Avoid the milkshakes in fast food restaurants.

Δ Get steamed veggies on the side.

Δ Opt for the plain baked potato (*not* the loaded baked potato) or the fruit cup.

LETTING IT ALL DIGEST

Along with breathing, eating is one of the activities we all must do to live. We must eat in order to live. Conversely, we mustn't live to eat, as the saying goes. That is one of the primary points of this chapter.

Healthy eating habits today are much different of days gone by. Healthy eating can and should be enjoyable and delicious. In many ways, it's also much easier. Steaming a scrumptious meal requires less effort in both preparation and clean-up than deep frying a grease-sodden catastrophe. And it also feels better.

When you eat well and properly, you, simply put, feel better. After a good meal, you feel full, yet light. Rather than feeling broadsided by gobs of fat and cholesterol, you feel the push of energy from the right foods impelling you to move.

Here's one thing you will notice as you shift your eating habits: once the shadows of flavors past are removed from your taste buds, you will begin to truly taste the deliciousness of properly and simply prepared foods: the snap of steamed and lightly-seasoned broccoli, the tang of briskly sautéed asparagus, the delicateness of a lightly baked fish.

Getting hungry? Good. With what you now know, you're ready to eat. And you might need it because in the next chapter, we're going to be moving.

Bon apetit!

7
MOVE YOUR BODY
YOU DON'T NEED A GYM TO WORKOUT

DO YOUR REMEMBER LEARNING TO RIDE A BIKE AS a child? Remember going outside to play with friends? Playing tag, freeze tag, or even "red light, green light"? What about sports or summer camp?

For many of us, being active in this way was a great source of fun and a way that our parents let us blow off steam. Then, one day, it all changed. As adults, we got caught up with work and began to see exercise as a chore rather than as play.

Movement is in our very nature, though! As children we loved to run, jump, and climb over various household (and sometimes non-household) objects. Even in our adulthood, our bodies have a constant and innate need for motion. We are constantly in motion whether we are aware of it or not: our hearts are beating; our lungs are taking in air; our nerves are firing; our eyes are blinking. If our bodies so desire that motion, why do we resist it so?

The most common excuse I hear is that there isn't any time. Due to work, family , children, or other commit-ments, there just aren't enough hours in the day to exercise.

Another excuse is that a gym membership is too expensive. Along with that, some people believe that exercising entails going to a gym—and they don't like gyms.

One other excuse I often hear is that some people just don't like exercising. Simple. And, at least they're honest.

The bottom line of all these excuses is that exercising just isn't a priority for many people. Getting through the barriers of exercise just means getting past the semantics of what exercise is.

WHAT IS EXERCISE?

When we get caught up with the word exercise, it really makes it seem like a chore. Additionally, we hear so much about how we "have to" exercise. It's a part of human nature that we resist doing those things that we "have to" do.

So, what really is exercise? At it's heart, unless you're training for the Olympics or are a professional athlete, exercise is just an activity that you do that elevates your baseline vitals (heart rate, blood pressure, breath rate) and expends energy. Essentially, it's just fun movement.

Isn't that less daunting? It doesn't seem like much of a chore now, does it?

As a "fun movement," exercise can be almost any physical activity that you enjoy on a regular basis. The physical activity could be anything from gardening to dancing. If you enjoy sports, exercise can be flag football, softball, basketball, volleyball, even kickball. You may enjoy hiking, biking, skiing, skating, or roller blading. There are a lot of middle-aged and elderly people that I know that love to go for a walk in a mall. Even running around with your children can get your heart rate up! (I have a good friend who lost over fifteen pounds just running after her toddler.) As a matter of fact, with many of today's gaming systems, you can build a sweat with games such as tennis, kickboxing, dancing, and even yoga in the comfort of your own home.

Get out your notebook. (You might have to get up and move to do that. Good for you!) Here's your first step toward moving towards a fun active lifestyle. Make a list of thirty things that you like to do that are active. If you don't know what you like to do, think about what interests you or what you'd like to try.

EVERYDAY EXERCISE IDEAS

Following our definition of exercise—"fun movement"—you can easily see how you can turn everyday activities into mini workout sessions. Here are some ideas.

Take the stairs. Take the stairs instead of taking the elevator (or escalator) when you are out. If there are stairs in your work place, you might even take a break to have a brisk walk up and down a couple of flights just to get the heart rate up a bit.

Park far away from the stores. Instead of wasting time and gasoline riding through the parking lot stalking people for a prime parking spot, park further away and enjoy a brisk walk to the door. It may not be much, but these small steps add up over the course of the day, a week, and a lifetime.

Mall walking. A 30-minute walk through the mall is more interesting than an outdoor track or a gym treadmill. Bonus: it's warmer in the winter. At the end of your walk, reward yourself with a little shopping or, depending on your mall, maybe a treat from the juice bar.

Dance. Whether you are in a class learning a routine, at a dance social, at a club, or at home in your living room, dancing is a fun way to slim down. If you are not a stellar dancer, turn on your favorite music in the privacy of your own home and just move your body. No one will see or judge you.

Walk your dog. You gotta do it anyway, so you might as well enjoy it. Take your dog for a good walk before or after work. Our pets need exercise, too. We are not the only beings suffering from obesity, diabetes, and heart failure. So if you won't do it for yourself, consider doing it for your little friend.

Turn on your TV. If you have cable, you will find that most companies have a "fitness channel." If not, then there are plenty of fitness DVDs you can buy. This can be a great alternative to a "formal" fitness class in a gym, especially if you haven't the time.

THE WILLINGNESS TO CHANGE

One thing is required to get some exercise in your daily life other than redefining it: a willingness and commitment to make the change. Recall from the process of change that planning and action come only after the commitment. While I can tell you the many benefits of exercise—how it lowers weight and blood pressure and increases metabolism and blood flow to the muscles and organs of the body; that it's good for lowering cholesterol and stabilizing the blood sugar; that physical activity helps to relieve stress and decreases anxiety and depression; that it will help you sleep better and works wonders for insomnia—the more important thing to understand is the effect that a life void of physical activity has on you *personally*. In order to demonstrate this, let's take an inventory.

Fill in the blanks of the following sentences.

A sedentary lifestyle causes my self-responsibility and self-esteem to be _____.

A sedentary lifestyle makes my breathing _____.

A sedentary lifestyle makes my senses _____.

A sedentary lifestyle affects my eating habits by _____.

A sedentary lifestyle causes me to feel _____.

A sedentary lifestyle makes my physical body _____.

A sedentary lifestyle makes my communication _____.

A sedentary lifestyle makes my thinking _____.

A sedentary lifestyle causes my work and play life to be _____.

A sedentary lifestyle makes my intimate or close relationships _____.

A sedentary lifestyle makes my ability to find meaning in life _____.

A sedentary lifestyle makes my connection with my higher source _____.

You may find that a sedentary lifestyle does not affect every one of these dimensions. The point of the exercise is to see how not being physically active on a regular basis can affect *many* areas of your life.

Let's flip this to the positive and look at the benefits that might come out of being active more regularly.

Regular physical activity affects my self-responsibility and self-esteem by _____.

Regular physical activity causes my breathing to be _____.

Regular physical activity causes my senses to be _____.

Regular physical activity affects my eating by _____.

Regular physical activity causes me to feel _____.

Regular physical activity causes my physical body to be _____.

Regular physical activity makes my communication _____.

Regular physical activity causes makes my thoughts _____.

Regular physical activity causes my work and play life to be _____.

Regular physical activity makes my intimate or close relationships _____.

Regular physical activity makes my ability to find meaning in life _____.

Regular physical activity makes my connection with my higher source _____.

Reflect on how your life is affected by your own choice to either be active or stay sedentary. You are your body's keeper. That means that the responsibility of your health is largely yours. Owning that responsibility by checking your attitude and being willing to take the first step gives you more power to step into a greater authentic and more free you, which results in health and wellness.

STAYING MOTIVATED

Once you get started with exercising, you will want to keep going. Unfortunately, sometimes life interrupts and you'll find yourself "just taking a day off." That's when it becomes very tempting to take two, then three, then the next thing you know, you're sedentary once again.

So, how to you stay on track? Here are four effective ways to keep yourself moving.

Do fun stuff. If you like what you're doing, you look forward to doing it, so incorporate more fun activities into your active life. Remember that exercise is simply "fun movement." When you make it fun, you'll keep doing it.

Get a partner. Having a group or a partner or a "workout buddy" always makes it more fun and it keeps you accountable.

Change your attitude. Again, we get caught up in the semantics of what exercise has to be. If you make it fun and you change your outlook to "I get to" instead of "I have to," you're more likely to be motivated to get out there are be active.

Set a goal. Some people are more goal-motivated than others. If that describes you, then set a goal (or a few goals) for yourself and don't stop until you reach it (or them). Your goal can be as simple as a weight-loss target or as complex as committing to walking a certain amount per week. The nice (and fun) thing about having exercise goals is that they put you in a competition—where your opponent is yourself.

8
THOUGHTS BECOME THINGS
YOUR ATTITUDE MATTERS

EVER WONDER WHY PEOPLE WHO COMPLAIN ARE always unhappy? Or why some people can always get what they want? Do you wonder why people who say they're always sick are always sick? Why people who claim to have bad luck usually do? What do you think the common denominator is? What if I told you that it's probably that they don't take responsibility for their own thoughts and feelings?

Are you aware that every thought is processed and integrated physically into your body, into your spirit, and into your world? Take a moment right now. What's on your mind? Write it down. What messages are you sending? Are they positive? Are they negative? Are they filled with fear and self-doubt? Or confidence and gratitude?

Most people aren't conscious of the thoughts that run through their heads. You may not even realize that your thoughts create feelings that cycle into more thoughts.

But you have a choice in your thinking. Just like when you drive a car you can decide where you want to go and then steer in any direction, you, too, can steer your thoughts and go in any direction you wish.

A Small Shift in Thinking

Here is an example of how just a small shift in thinking changed my actions—and therefore changed the world around me.

The year that I was writing this book was a particularly challenging for me. There were a lot of new things happening and plenty of roadblocks. I consistently practiced gratitude by getting up every morning and writing five things down for which I was grateful. Well, that summer, I began to notice that my attitude was more negative than usual. I was complaining more and I was just not feeling like things were moving forward for me. I still got up every morning and wrote my gratitude list and read my daily inspirational readings, but things still felt off. So I started to re-listening to some of my mentors, the people who have inspired me and helped to keep me on my path. I was listening to a podcast done by my good friend Antonio, who has been integral to many of my breakthroughs during the year. He said, "If you're going to be grateful, really be grateful. Really feel the gratitude in your body, in every cell. Jump up and down as if it were the first time that you ever saw Christmas day! I mean, just be excited." At that moment, it clicked for me. During my gratitude sessions, I was just going through the motions: I was just writing down things for which I was grateful and not really feeling them. I was reading my inspirational messages just from rote practice. So at that moment I made the choice that I would get excited about every gratitude list that I wrote and really feel it. Let me tell you, when I started doing that I immediately felt multiple shifts—a shift in my attitude, a shift in my thinking, and a shift in the world around me. Things began to change, everything falling right into sync just as if God had said, "That's what I was waiting for." It was a great lesson that the way I think really does affect my outside world. It wasn't just my perception; what I was putting out there was coming right back to me.

Can you think of a time when your attitude—good or bad—brought you exactly what you sent? Think of a situation where you may have had an opportunity to approach something from a positive angle, but you chose to play the blame game, or victim role. Be very honest with yourself. Journal and reflect about how your negative attitude might have (or actually) affected your outcome.

Mental Chatter

Have you ever noticed that you don't hear too many five-year-olds contemplating, "Mommy, what if I don't make the soccer team?" or "Daddy, what if I don't fit into those jeans from last year?" That's because kids are too busy living in the moment, so their thoughts don't go there. They only begin to think those thoughts after they've had several external messages telling them that they are not good enough as they are. We need to make sure that we watch what we say around our children because it has lasting effects.

Likewise, we need to watch what we say to ourselves.

We all have our own mental chatter. It's the dialogue that goes on in your head when you're not focused on one thing or another—when you're zoning out. Realize, though, that your thoughts—even those "unfocused," chatty thoughts—are powerful and creative. The things you think about you bring about. Your thoughts become your perceptions; they create feelings about yourself and others.

Consider your own mental chatter. What subtle messages are you sending yourself? Let's take a thoughts inventory. As you do this, make a mental note of how your thoughts today have affected the other dimensions of your wellness.

EXERCISE: THOUGHTS INVENTORY

How have your thoughts reflected or affected your self-responsibility?

How have they affected your self-love?

How have your thought processes affected your breathing?

Your senses?

Have your thoughts affected your eating?

Have they affected how you feel today?

How have your thought processes affected your communication?

Your moving?

How have your thoughts affected your work day? Or your ability to relax and play?

Have your thoughts today affected your intimate or close relationships?

How do they affect your ability to find meaning in life?

How do they affect your relationship or your communication with your higher power?

MESSAGES TO YOURSELF

Let's talk about some of the negative and positive messages you may be giving yourself. Do you—or does anyone you know—constantly make any of these statements:

I'm always getting sick.

I'm too broke for that.

I hate my job.

I give up.

If only this would happen, then that would be better.

I am always tired.

I never get enough sleep.

I don't have time for me.

There aren't enough hours in the day.

I don't make friends easily.

You can't trust anyone.

I'm such an idiot!

I should know better.

I could never be _____.

I'm always stressed out.

I feel like I'm getting old.

While subtle, these statements send a deeper message to your inner psyche that both support and create the negative space that you're in. What are some other examples that I may not have listed here of negative dialogue that you or someone else you know may be sending?

Conversely, making positive statements send a similar message to create positive feelings, actions, or situations. That's why gratitude works so well.: it reinforces in your mind the good that you have in life. Here are some positive statements that you may have heard people make. Have you noticed that they are usually right on target?

I can eat whatever I want and never gain weight.

I just don't get sick.

I always have enough money.

I have so much free time to do what I want.

I have a super immune system.

I'm human, so it's okay that I make mistakes sometimes.

I just age well.

I love what I do.

I pretty much get along with everyone.

It is what it is.

My intuition never lies.

I have so much energy all the time.

I always sleep like a baby.

I'm in the best shape of my life.

I feel ten years younger than I really am.

Stop here for a minute and write down some of the things that you say to yourself, both positive and negative. Then write what messages you may be sending that might be creating your very reality.

Remember when we talked about treating your body like the temple that it is? Your thoughts and self-talk is a way you treat yourself—and they can (and usually do) affect your health and wellness.

Take for example worry and stress, two common things of which there is far too much in our lives today. Worry and stress causes a baseline inflammation in your body, which is the basis of many diseases and disorders. Thoughts of worry and stress can contribute to all of the following conditions[1]:

Obesity   *Diabetes*   *Stomach ulcers*
Irritable bowel syndrome   *Erectile dysfunction*
Migraine headaches   *High blood pressure*

BOB AND MANNY (EXAMPLE)

Bob and Manny have the same job at the same level of pay. They work the same hours under the same boss and have the same deadlines. They're both married with two children.

Bob has hypertension and irritable bowel syndrome[2]. He's constantly stressed about deadlines, often skips lunch, and frequently complains that he's tired because he can never get enough sleep. One day at lunch, he even confided to Manny that he and his wife were having problems because he was so stressed at work and that he was coming home more irritable and preoccupied with what he had going on that today.

Manny, who was a very healthy, happily married man, gently counseled his friend that one thing that may help is if he left work at work. That way he could appreciate the time with his wife and children when

---

1 It can even affect the severity of course of conditions like lupus, sickle cell, and various cancers. Naturally, stress and worry can also contribute to mental disorders such as panic attacks, insomnia, anxiety, depression, and acute stress reactions.

2 Also known as "spastic colon," Irritable Bowel Syndrome (IBS) presents with chronic abdominal pain, bloating, and irregular bowel habits. It's cause is unknown.

he came home. He even suggested that Bob take his wife out on a date so that they could reconnect to the young people they both fell in love with in the first place.

These two simple things were just the motivation Bob needed to start looking at his behavior. He went home that night and asked his wife out on a date. When she showed loving surprise and said yes, he embraced her with a kiss and they both slept well that night. The next morning Bob was refreshed. He faced work with more vigor and confidence because he had something to look forward to this weekend. He thanked his friend Manny and vowed to begin making some changes in his life.

Over time Bob began working out, eating healthier, and, eventually, he was able to come off the blood pressure medicine and his irritable bowel syndrome subsided. It only took a little motivation from a friend and an open mind to change his thinking for Bob to turn his life in a totally different direction.

While that story may strike you as a little dramatic, it is based on true people and true event. Time and again I have seen one thought making a huge difference in a person's life. Consider how your thoughts affect your feelings about relationships. You've heard the phrase "taking the plunge" when people talk about marriage, I am sure. Don't you think these three little words reveal a dismal attitude towards marriage? If you take this approach to marriage, it seems only natural that the marriage would be destined to fail. Looking at the divorce rates, you'd have to agree that there's something to this. Have you ever seen those couples who have been happily married for 30, 40 or even 50 years? They don't view marriage as a prison sentence; they view it as a partnership. These people are best friends and each person allows the other the freedom to be themselves. What is the difference in their attitude toward their marriage and toward their partner? Your attitude matters—and your attitude begins with your thoughts.

A VICIOUS CYCLE

I had an interesting conversation with a good friend about a year ago. I was newly dating at the time and I was sharing my dating experiences with her. As we compared experiences, I noticed that my experiences were positive while she seemed to be having trouble meeting someone that suited her. As I listened to her, I noticed that all of her statements about men were negative: she complained about how good men seemed to be so hard to find and that she felt like she would never find a man. I, on the other hand, had met quite a few very nice men. I explained to my friend that if she continued to have the attitude that there were no good men left or that she would never find a good man, then that would continue to be her experience. I have never subscribed to the statement that "all men are dogs" and I have always believed that there is a good man out there for everyone.

Stereotyping, such as what my friend was doing, creates a cycle that encourages the object being generalized to act, at least to your perception, in the way that they are expected to. Take the state of the economy at any given time. Your stereotyping of it can create a cycle that can bring about the fear that you express. If you become afraid because you think that "times are bad" and it's "really rough out there," then you'll stop buying things, which will affect businesses as they lose sales and revenue, which in turn will affect you as you lose hours or even get laid off. From thought to reality. A cycle is created. Talk about a self-fulfilling prophecy! All of this from the collective thought of a society—which is comprised of individuals' thoughts.

But I'm sure you think that your thoughts and collective thoughts have nothing to do with it. I mean, it really *is* bad out there, right?

YOUR FEELINGS

As we look at our thoughts, we can't ignore our feelings because they are very much intertwined. As you've seen, your negative thoughts can create fears that can produce a vicious cycle that comes back to reflect and reinforce our feelings and affect our actions. Your feelings affect your relationships and your environment and are a result of how you think and how you communicate. In fact, we often let our feelings rule our actions and control our lives. It all comes back to the language we use in our self-talk.

Have you ever noticed how honest children are about their feelings? They have a very acute awareness of their feelings and they say exactly what they mean. Children are the essence of authenticity. However, as children experience the world, they learn to hide and lie about their emotions. They also learn to be controlled by their feelings. Consider that as a child, when you experienced an emotion, you didn't let it affect the next action. You experienced it, then went on about your life once the experience passed. It isn't until other people (adults, media, other children) give meaning to the experience of the emotion making it have a lasting effect on our future experiences.

Let's check in with ourselves right now. How are you feeling at *this* moment? Think of some specific feeling words to describe how you're feeling, not just "good" or "bad." Be more specific. Are you feeling depressed? Are you feeling elated? Are you feeling excited? Are you feeling motivated? Are you feeling deceived? Are you feeling tired? Are you feeling angry? Are you feeling fearful? Are you feeling rested? Are you feeling relaxed? Are you feeling lovable? Are you feeling accepted? Are you feeling cared about? All of these different things are ways that you can be feeling. Now think about how you feel. How is this affecting your day today? What meaning are you bringing to your feelings? How is it affecting the rest of the dimensions that we've mentioned earlier?

FEELINGS INVENTORY

How do your feelings affect your self-responsibility?
How have your feelings affected your self-love?
Your breathing?
Your senses?
How have your feelings affected your eating?

What about your thinking?

How have they affected your communication?

Have they affected how much you moved today?

How much you've played today?

Have they affected your work dimension?

Your close relationships?

Your working relationships?

How do your feelings affect your ability to find meaning in life?

How do your feelings affect your relationship with your higher power?

This is an exercise you can do any time and I'd like to challenge you to do the following: Check in with your feelings as you are with your thoughts at least once a day. When you do this check in, notice what meaning are you bringing to your feelings and how that meaning is affecting your reality. Also notice whether your thought process contributed to your present feeling and vice versa. Are you in a vicious cycle?

BREAKING THE CYCLE

Let's talk about how to break that cycle. There are many ways that you can change your mental chatter when you're having a day not to your liking. One of the best ways is shifting your internal dialogue. And there are many ways to accomplish that.

Declarations. Mentioned earlier in this book, declarations are very important in creating your reality. Declarations are positive statements in the present tense that bring a possibility forth into being. Declarations are best made daily and with enthusiasm.[3] Declarations have no power without action behind them, though. Larry Pearson, one of my coaches, said, "There are two tongues in the body: the one in the mouth and the one in the shoe—and the one in the shoe never lies." In other words, talk is cheap unless it is backed by action.

Gratitude. Starting your day with gratitude can shift your view of the day and help you to see the possibilities already in front of you—and some that don't even exist yet. You remember the example I gave you earlier of how when I really started to feel the gratitude my view of life shifted and thus did my experience. That's how gratitude works. Ending the day in gratitude helps you to complete and let go of anything that is not a clearing for power in your life. It can shift your immediate experience in any situation. Gratitude can also bring you to the present moment by replacing cycling or obsessive negative thought patterns.

Changing Your Self-Talk. Here's a fact: self-talk is a technique that is used all of the time in business, especially in the sales world. Why? Because it works. Positive self-talk is simply a self-declaration. When professionals prepare for a big presentation, they empower themselves with their self-talk by declaring the results that they *want*. Positive self-talk is simply shifting the context of the mind. It builds confidence. Managing your internal dialogue like this on a regular basis will greatly impact your sense of self-love and responsibility.

Try this exercise: Each morning when you wake up, look

---

3 You may even use a vision board, which is a note board that you hang on your wall onto which you post pictures and images of your goals.

in your mirror—straight in the eye—and decalre, "Who I am is powerful, peaceful, and prodcutive! Who I am is beautiful and magnetic! Who I am is supported and loved!"

What will this accomplish (other than making you feel silly at first)? You will be creating a brand new you! Each morning as you create yourself newly, you will begin to feel a shift in your being; you will begin to take on these ways of being naturally.[4]

Along with your self-talk, each morning when you wake up, give yourself a big hug.[5] Then you can tell yourself you love yourself and how good you look and that you're good enough. For the record, if you already have self-esteem, this exercise doesn't hurt at all.

This is not about creating "feel good moments." It's about creating a completely new way of being that becomes a way of life. As you transform your thought processes, you transform you way of being. From this transformation, you have the ability to live and act from a place of authentic power. Can you imagine how this would impact your life? Can you imagine how being in this power would impact others?

SHIFTING CONTEXT WITH DECLARATIONS

As you've seen, declarations, positive or negative, create yourself and your world. It is imperative, then, to create and use positive declarations rather than negative ones.

---

4 As with any practice, consistency is key; if you do not do this exercise consistently, the results disappear, if any come at all.

5 Did you know that studies have found that a person should get sixteen hugs per day? Human contact via hugs reduces stress and reinforces the feeling of interconnectedness a person should have. It promotes both mental and physical health.

First, you must become aware of when you are talking to yourself negatively. At first, this might be somewhat difficult. As you practice and get in tune with yourself, this will become easier and easier. How often can or do you catch yourself in negative thought? When you become good at this, you may then start countering these negative statements with positive declarations. Basically, you're beginning to retrain the brain, shifting its usual default way of being to a space of new possibility.

For example, if you find yourself thinking,

"I can't believe I did that."

You can counter that with,

"I'm human and sometimes mistakes happen."

Here are more examples.

Negative: "I can't afford _____."
Counter: "It only seems like I cannot afford this; I can create abundance in my life whenever I choose."

Negative: "I can't do this."
Counter: "It only seems like it is hard; I can do anything."

Negative: "What's wrong with me?"
Counter: "I am perfect, whole, and complete."

Negative: "I have to get this done."
Counter: "I will get this done, no problem! Who I am is super-productive!"

Negative: "I'm too fat."
Counter: "I am beautiful."

Become aware of the negative thoughts that you have about yourself or that you say to yourself. Create counter declarations for them. This is a very good exercise to do and I challenge you to start doing it today. At least once a day become aware of your thoughts; then, at least once a day, catch yourself and counter it with a positive declaration aloud.

POSITIVE ACTION

Another way to shift yourself out of a negative thought process or a negative feeling is distraction by positive action. Let me give you two examples of how these tools have worked with former clients. Let's call them Mary and Mike.

Mary is feeling stress about her finances. She begins obsessing about how she's going to pay her bills. Although she has a solid job and is a valuable member of her company and is not likely to get laid off, she has seen many of her colleagues go so she constantly worries about being let go as well. She feels an anxiety attack coming on. She immediately picks up the phone and calls a friend that she knows is going through a tough divorce and asks her how she is doing and proceeds to just listen. Mary takes herself out of her own negative and obsessive thoughts and dedicates herself to a positive action to someone else.

Did you ever notice that people who are happy and successful also happen to do a lot of volunteer work? Do you think the success came before the volunteer work? Or did the volunteer work follow the success? Chances are likely that you will find that it is the former rather than the latter. Why? Helping people feels good. Again, why? Because it reinforces within us the notion that we are worthy and that we have a place—a meaning— in life. In Mary's case, while she wasn't saving the world, she was using her time to help her friend. Just the act of her being a support for her friend helped her to realize her usefulness and her value.

Here's another example.

Mike and his wife have been having marital difficulties of late. He is on his way home from work anticipating the fight that he knows is going to happen because he had to stay an hour late at work. He can just hear the conversation in his head and the resulting tension that will carry throughout the rest of the evening. He becomes tense and angry just at the thought of it. Suddenly, his cell phone rings; it's his friend. As he talks to his friend, he realizes how ridiculous his non-existent "argument" with his wife is and jokingly mentions it to his friend. He then listen as his friend offers some encouragement and then lends an understanding ear.

Mike's distraction served as a shift to the imagined experience he was playing in his head. That distraction snapped him back to reality, so to speak. How many times has this happened to you? How many times have you been caught up in your mental world—either positive or negative—only to be brought back to reality by something?

These are two purposely small examples to illustrate how easily we can get lost in our thoughts and how just small, seemingly insignificant positive actions either of our own accord or brought upon us by others can shift our thoughts from a negative space to a positive one. Thus, the key is that if you find yourself in a negative thought space, then you should make a positive action. Snap yourself back to reality! Realize that what you're thinking isn't real.

Finally, continue to take personal inventory of your thoughts. Remember that change is a process. Years of thinking one way will not change in one week, one day, or even one month. It can take years. So be patient and gentle with yourself. Remember, awareness, acceptance, and action.

NEGATIVE INTO POSITIVE EXERCISES

Create your own declarations. Now is the time to really get busy. Make your declarations in the present tense. Make it affirm a particular goal or desire. Repeat it daily first thing in the morning.

A-to-Z gratitude exercise. Go through the alphabet from the letter A to Z and with every letter name something that you're grateful for.

Five things a day gratitude list. Write five things that you're grateful for each morning before you even get out of the bed. Notice how this shapes your days, your weeks, and your months. Don't believe me? Make a commitment to do this for thirty days. See what happens.

Positive sublimation. Think of some positive actions that can help you get out of your "stinkin' thinkin'." Make a list of those actions for those moments of mental distress. It's always good to be prepared.

YOUR THOUGHTS AND YOUR WELLNESS

You might be asking yourself right now *What does all this thought stuff have to do with my health and wellness?*

Have you heard of the Placebo Effect? Doctors and researchers have found that in some cases, when patients were purposely given ineffective or fake medication, the patients responded as if they had taken effective or real medication and showed actual improvement. For example, a patient who suffered from frequent headaches was given sugar pills by his doctor. Even though the pills should not have had any effect, they did and the patient ceased having frequent headaches.

While researches are uncertain why this happens, one theory is that there most certainly is a mind-body connection and as you think (or, more importantly, *believe*) something to be true you tend to actualize it in your experience. Thus, because our headache sufferer believed that he was taking proper medication on orders from a proper doctor, he "believed" himself well in the process.

Now, I'm not saying that a person can believe their cancer away. What I am saying is that you have greater control over your health and wellness than you imagine. And it all begins with your thoughts—about yourself and about your world around you.

In the simplest sense, your thoughts (which include thoughts about yourself and others, your perceptions, and your beliefs) produce your feelings (everything from love and acceptance to fear and worry) which then produce your actions (from the good to the bad to even your non-action). The actions that you take then mold and shape your environment and your relationships. Everything is interconnected and intertwined.

You awaken every morning with a smile and greet yourself with positivity and respect. This builds self-love and confidence within you, which then enables you to meet new people and make new friends. When the time comes that things are getting shaky at work, you don't worry; instead you network with your friends asking them if they know of any openings. A few of your friends respond positively and before you know it you have a new and better position. This not only saves you from the "wear and tear" of worry; it also allows you to not have to scrimp and cut back and you can keep buying the good food choices that help you stay healthy and well.

See? One thing leads to another. In a house or a building, if one board or girder was not in place or is defective in some way, then the building would collapse.

It's the same thing with your life and your health and wellness. Each step—each facet—is an integral part of your entire wellness system without which you run the risk of falling into not-wellness.

That's why it is imperative that you follow this Wellness Blueprint.

That's why it's imperative that you watch your thoughts.

PART III

STRUCTURE

He who has health, has hope; and he who has hope, has everything.

—Thomas Carlyle

9
BOUNDARIES AND BALANCE
WORK, PLAY, REST, LIFE

IT'S EASY TO GET CAUGHT UP IN YOUR WORK EN-vironment so much so that you forget to take time to play. It's easy to forget to take down time for yourself. It's easy to overlook that life is not just all about working and making a living. In this chapter we're going to talk about balancing your work and your fun. We're also going to balance both of those with rest and downtime.[1] In short, along with reclaiming your health and wellness, you're also going to reclaim your life.

BOUNDARIES

Let's start with work. What happens if there's too much work and no play? You become irritable, resentful, bored, and even stressed. Here's another question: Do you love what you do at work? Do you have fun at work? It's important to remember that work can be fun as well, but how do you do this? How do you balance the stressors at work with fun? How do you incorporate playfulness into your work environment?

---

1 I've found that even people who balance their work and their play often forget about rest and downtime, both of which are important to your overall wellness. We'll be addressing that as well.

You might not believe this now, but it's really just as simple as making the decision to do so. You're going to do this—and you're going to see why it is easier than you think—in the framework of boundaries.

What is a **boundary**? The definition of boundary is "a limit of a subject or sphere of activity." Sometimes, to truly understand the meaning of something, it helps to look at the effects of that something. So let's look at what happens when boundaries break down.

When you don't apply boundaries at work, you end up overworked and (potentially) burned out. This can have a negative effect on interaction with your family.

What happens when we don't set limits with our family and children? We can end up neglecting and perhaps not taking care of the basic things like proper nutrition or exercise or even having quiet time with ourselves.

What about society and values? When we don't place a limit on ourselves or on society, we can end up compromising who we are just to fit in.

And what about when we don't set limits or boundaries with ourselves? We over commit, we can become ill, and we can get burned out. Overall, we can become very dis-empowered and out of control.

With those negative effects of not having boundaries in mind, what are some of the reasons that we do not set boundaries?

Sometimes setting them seems selfish. (You may be used to doing things for other people, but there is a difference between selfishness and self-care.)

Some people just don't know how to set boundaries. If you grew up in a household where no limits were set or if you grew up in a household where your limits were constantly violated, this can leave you not knowing how to set boundaries or even not knowing how to be able to hold the boundaries that you place for others and yourself.

Sometimes we don't set boundaries for fear of hurting someone else. Have you ever stayed in a relationship longer than you wanted because you didn't want to hurt the other person's feelings? Have you ever picked up the slack at work because you just couldn't bring yourself to tell a colleague that their work needed improvement?

Sometimes we don't set boundaries because of the fear of someone being angry with us. A work colleague asks you to stay late and help him with a project; you stay late and miss your son's baseball game because you're afraid of the repercussions of your colleague being angry with you. This also relates to the reason of wanting people to like us (or being afraid that people won't like us) if we set those limits and boundaries.

The truth about boundaries is this: **setting boundaries and limits is healthy for not only yourself but for the person that you're setting the limit for.** Boundaries affect your safety, your sanity, your security, and your stress levels. Remember when we talked about self-responsibility and what happens when there's over-responsibility? When there's over responsibility we tend not to set boundaries. And when you don't set boundaries, you begin to assume responsibility for things you shouldn't. That, of course, leads to problems. See how everything intertwines and integrates with each other?

WHAT'S YOURS AND WHAT'S NOT

Let's talk about the what's yours and what's not yours. Your issues are your awareness of your inner life. This includes your beliefs, thoughts, feelings, decisions, choices, experiences, wants and needs, and your unconscious material. It also includes your own behavior. The responsibility to make your life successful and joyful is solely yours. This means that other people's awareness of their own inner life—their beliefs, thoughts, feelings, decisions, choices, experiences, wants and needs, and unconscious materials as well as behaviors—are *their* issues and not yours.

Let's do a quick exercise. I want you to decide whether or not each scenario is *your stuff* or *somebody else's stuff*. The answers will be given after the examples.

1. Your sister gets evicted from her apartment because of poor decisions she has made and asks you to move all of her furniture at the last minute.

2. Your feelings are hurt because your boss offers you some constructive criticism and you believe that you are being picked on.

3. Your mom asked to borrow some money to pay her bills because she frivolously spent her money on new furniture this month.

4. Your significant other hesitates to answer the question of whether you should come over and you interpret that they must be hiding something.

5. You share a concern with your friend about a change in your work schedule and she immediately tells you what you should be doing since she has gone through this before.

If you said for number one that it's your sister's issues and not yours, you are correct. Your sister's poor decisions are not your issue and, at this point, you would have the right to set a limit if you are not willing to move that furniture at the last minute for fun and for free. You would be well within your domain.

For number two, if your feelings are hurt because of your perception that you're being picked on, that's your stuff. That's your issue and that's your perspective, because you don't know whether your boss is trying to pick on you or not.

If your mother is asking for money, as in number three, because she made the decision to frivolously spend her money on something else, that's her responsibility, not yours.

In number four, your interpretation that your significant other may be hiding something is definitely your stuff and not theirs. Even if there has been some dishonesty in the past, this is still your perception. That is not to say that it's not a valid feeling, but if you're making the choice to stay with someone who's dishonest, then whose stuff is that? (Hint: All yours.)

For number five, if you're sharing a concern with a friend and they begin to tell you what to do based on what they've gone through, that's definitely not your stuff. You have choices and you get to make the decisions based on what you feel and think—not based on what somebody else has been through. If you choose to take their advice, that's okay; just make sure that you understand that you are basing your decision on what you trust from someone else's experiences.

Can you think of any other situations that you might have experienced where you have to distinguish your stuff from someone else's?

SETTING HEALTHY BOUNDARIES

Before we go on to apply setting limits to our work, our home, our family, and our play, let's set some healthy criteria for setting boundaries.

First, you have to be present. If you're not aware that the limit needs to be set, then you're not able to set it. Seems simple, but you'd be surprised at how many people think that working through lunch is perfectly normal.

Second, the boundary has to be appropriate. As was noted earlier, a boundary has to be based on *your* issues, *your* inner life, *your* thoughts, *your* beliefs, *your* feelings—and not on the issues of others.

Third, the boundary needs to be protective. It should be used to *protect* your well-being and not to hurt or punish or control others. Not helping a friend because of a perceived (on your part) injustice is different than not helping because it's unworkable for you. One is a form of revenge (some might call it "passive aggressiveness"), the other is being conscious of each other's responsibilities.

Fourth, the boundary needs to be clear. Before you set the boundary, be clear about what the boundary is. When you're clear about it with yourself, you can effectively communicate it to others. For example, if I'm clear that I need more sleep, I can't just say "I'm going to go to bed earlier"; that's not clear. A clear limit may be, "I want to sleep more, so I'm going to start going to bed by 10:30 p.m., which means all phone calls need to stop by 10 p.m." This way I can communicate a clear boundary to my friends and family, in this case that unless there's an emergency, please do not call my home phone after 10.

Fifth, the boundary needs to be firm. If the boundary is not firm, then the limit is less effective, if it is at all. For example, I asked my family that unless it's an emergency, please don't call my home phone after 10 p.m. When the phone rings at 10:15 and I'm in the bed, I might need to reinforce that by saying, "Hi, you know I'm in bed, can you call me back tomorrow if it's not an emergency?" By reinforcing this boundary, you're making it firm so that it can be respected in the future. When people know that you're very serious about a boundary, they tend to respect it.

Sixth, the boundary must be maintained. In keeping with the example of the phone, if I set the limit that I don't want people to call my home phone after 10 p.m., yet a few nights a week I'm making calls to others at 10:30 or 11 p.m., then that's not maintaining the boundary and it undermines the credibility of the limit that you set in the first place.

Finally, the boundary needs to be flexible. The difference between a boundary and a rigid wall is that the boundary is flexible. When I set the phone boundary, I included an exception: "unless it's an emergency." So, if someone calls to tell me that my sister is in the hospital and it's after my boundary time, I'm not going to say, "I asked you not to call me after ten! I'll call you tomorrow." That would be very rigid. I know that's an extreme example, but it's an example of the difference between a wall and a boundary.

WORK BOUNDARIES

Now you know about setting limits. You know the guidelines, you know the difference between your issues and someone else's issues, and you know the indicators to set boundaries. Let's apply them to work.

Let's do a little exercise. Think of an instance from your past week where you could have set a boundary but you didn't. Think about the consequences of not having set that limit with your colleague or your coworker or your boss. What did it cost you? Emotional stress or strain? Time? Your lunch break?

What are some boundaries that you can set at work?

I just named one of them: eating lunch.[2] There are so many people that I know who work through lunch. It's very important to know that, just like a car, your body can't run on nothing. Food is the fuel that keeps you going. If you skip meals, just like a car, you'll run out of "gas" and you'll break down. So, can you set a limit to take fifteen to thirty minutes a day to eat lunch?

---

2 If you're a person who's always on the go, you may think about packing a sack lunch. Earlier in this book we talked about "brown-bagging it." We talked about snacks and lunches that are easy and portable. At this point, there's no excuse for missing a meal. This is all about changing your mindset and being willing to empower yourself so that you can be a healthier you.

What about the boundary of showing up to work on time? This is one that may make people say, "Huh?", But keep in mind that showing up for work on time is part of self-responsibility. It's a form of integrity. Remember that you're modeling—to children, to colleagues, to employees. If you consistently show up late, then it may give people permission to think that they can do the same thing. Showing up late to work may also be an indicator that you're either doing too much before work, not getting enough sleep the night before, or not being prepared enough to the morning of to get to work on time. Any of those may mean changing something in your household to set up proper support so that you can actually make it to work on time.

Likewise, leaving work on time is another important boundary to have in place. If you're used to working past the time that you're scheduled to leave work, begin setting a boundary for yourself to leave work as scheduled. See how much more time that will give you at home with your family.

If you're a small business owner or manager or in a profession where your work almost requires you to work off-hours, such as a lawyer, then you have two limits to set: the limit of when you're going to stop working *and* not bringing work home with you. The latter is a challenging one for a small business owner. (I admit that I'm guilty as charged. I sometimes find myself sitting in front of the television with my computer preparing for the next day of work.) I've found two boundaries useful for this tricky situation. The first is to set a time limit for working at home and, when I am working, I do my best to work distraction-free so that I am fully working and actually getting things done. The second boundary is to reserve one day as a "day of rest," where I only do work-related tasks in the case of an emergency or a pressing deadline, otherwise, I am off the clock. By creating those boundaries, I've found that I get more done when I work as I'm focused on working and not allowing myself to get distracted or interrupted.

What about setting the limit with yourself not take responsibility for other people's poor choices at work? Set the limit that you only help someone when it's for fun and for free, meaning you will not be resentful about it later.

Finally, what about the commitment that you'll insert some fun into your environment? How do you do that? It can be as simple as telling a joke, playing some good music, going to lunch with colleagues, or scheduling yourself a lunch date with your someone special. Try having a little office party just because. Take a moment and think of all the possibilities. How can you make your work fun and creative? Making work fun and creative is an important boundary to set because if you're going to be spending half of your waking day at work then you may as well like it.[3]

HOME AND FAMILY BOUNDARIES

You've worked all day and you come home to your family. Pow! There's a whole other responsibility there. You need to learn to set boundaries at home with your family just as well as you do with work.

---

3 If you don't like your work, then you should consider what you do like and move towards that in order to be in your authentic self.

Think about this: what happens when you don't say no at home? A lot of times, you continue to over-extend yourself, therefore never getting any time to yourself, which then leads to a whole array of stress and fatigue. Setting boundaries at home is just a form of taking care of yourself.

Here's an example of how not having boundaries affected a client of mine and how she resolved the situation. Jennifer was a successful corporate executive, wife and mother to two school-aged children. She was working ten-hour days before going home and immediately beginning dinner. She would help the children with their homework and then get them ready for bed. By the time she finished all this, she'd be exhausted and go straight to bed, only to wake up the next day and do the same thing again. On the weekends, her very active daughters played soccer and went to dance class, so she spent most of her Saturdays at practices, games, and dance recitals. When she came to me I asked her, "What do you do for fun and relaxation?" A confused look came over her face and it was apparent that there was no time for fun or relaxation for Jennifer.

What boundaries could Jennifer put in place to help her balance her family and her self-time? How could she lovingly approach her husband and her children to help her implement these boundaries and support her in holding them firm?

Here's what happened after Jennifer and I covered boundaries in our sessions: Jennifer called a family meeting and told her husband and children how exhausted she's been due to not having any down time. She explained that she would be implementing a "one hour after-work rule," which would give her one hour of quiet time immediately after work to "decompress." She asked her husband if he could take over helping the children with their homework; he agreed. Also, Jennifer suggested that once a month she and her husband get a babysitter and have a date night just for the two of them. Jennifer also asked for one Saturday night for just her so that she can either visit her girlfriends or even just have a quiet night to herself.

Thus, Jennifer's at-home boundaries were set. Now, this may not work so perfectly all the time, but it's an example of how you can engage your family into setting these boundaries.

PERSONAL BOUNDARIES

So far you've learned to set boundaries at home and at work. It's also important to set boundaries with yourself—of making *yourself* a priority. We touched on this briefly: not skipping lunch, leaving work on time, and making your health a priority. Let's go into it deeper with some specifics.

Eating. Make sure you're eating regularly, three to five small meals a day.

Sleep. I was on a radio show discussing how sleep is a time for regeneration and recharging and most people these days are only sleeping four to six hours a day, which is ridiculous. Thus, all of these disorders from stress and sleep deprivation, like anxiety or hypertension or even both, are starting to become quite prevalent. Make sure that you get six to eight hours of sleep a day.

Playtime. Do you regularly schedule time to do fun things in your life? to play? It's funny: we teach our children how to balance work with play, then we forget how to play ourselves! Frankly, it seems that our society is teaching (and modeling) work over play. Look at the emphasis on test scores in the schools and look at how they're taking the arts and sports and physical education out of the schools. This is sending a message to our children that play is not important, that it's not a priority, and that work is the highest (if not the only) priority. This is dysfunctional; we need to be careful because our society is already a high stress society with depression and anxiety being on the rise.[4] We as individual families and as a society need to watch our dialogue with and the examples we present to our children. We are essentially teaching imbalance to our children and by doing this we are walking on a slippery slope.[5]

I commonly see patients for stress and anxiety in my office. When I ask them what they do for fun, I am usually met with a blank stare. Now, we're all grown ups and we're all responsible, for all the grown-up things in life, but we're also responsible for our fun. So, let's look at how you can integrate play into your daily life. (I bet you know where

---

4 Childhood depression and anxiety are on the rise and show no indication of slowing and a significant factor of that rise is the importance placed on tests and test performance. This then creates a feedback loop whereby these conditions cause lowered test performance. If you get anything from this book, get the notion that everything is connected with one aspect affecting all the others.

5 Attention Deficit Hyperactivity Disorder (ADHD) is already an over-diagnosed condition for our children. Because of this often mis-diagnosed condition, substance abuse is on the rise as the children are being prescribed mood-altering drugs such as Ritalin, to which the children are then getting addicted.

I'm going with this. It's time for another inventory!)

Here's the question to ask yourself: What happens when there is no fun in your life?

When there is no fun in my life, my self-responsibility is _____.

When there is no fun in my life, my breathing is _____.

When there is no fun in my life, my senses are _____.

When there is no fun in my life, my eating is _____.

When there is no fun in my life, my feeling is _____.

When there is no fun in my life, my thinking is _____.

When there is no fun in my life, my communicating is _____.

When there is no fun in my life, my moving is _____.

When there is no fun in my life, my playing is _____.

When there is no fun in my life, my working is _____.

When there is no fun in my life, my intimate and close relationships are _____.

When there is no fun in my life, my ability to find meaning in life is _____.

When there is no fun in my life, my relationship with my higher power is _____.

Now do the same exercise with this sentence:

When I include fun and play in my life, my self-responsibility, breathing, sensing, eating, feeling, thinking, communicating, moving, playing, working, intimate and close relationships, ability to find meaning in life, relationship with my higher power, are _____.

Compare the two. Can you see the importance of scheduling time for play?

Finally, for those people who have worked so hard for so long that they have forgotten what they even like to do for fun or play, here's an exercise for you to discover that "spark" and rediscover yourself.

Make a **bucket list**. Yes, just like the movie of the same name, make a check list of about thirty things that you'd either like to do or have always wanted to do. Then, go about doing them one-by-one and checking them off the list. There's no time limit nor are there any "wrong" answers. Your list can include anything from painting a picture to learning to tango; they can be learning experiences or physical activities. Let your mind wander, don't hold back, and, if I may be a bit cliché, let your "inner child" run free.

There's no time like the present to include fun into your life. Life is too short. You must seize the day in a healthy way.

DOWNTIME

You're balancing your work and your home life. You're having fun. You're less stressed. There's just one more thing to attend to: quiet time or down time.

One of the things that I am always working towards is being able to balance activity with non-activity. Downtime is a must. It allows your body the opportunity to recharge and renew itself.

For the busy bees out there who work and play so much that they wear themselves out, do this: During the week, take two days and schedule *absolutely nothing* for the evening. That means you are scheduled to do nothing, not that you haven't planned anything. So, if someone asks you to do something after work, you say, "I'm busy." If they ask doing what, you say you're "busy doing nothing." Then you bring yourself home and you sit yourself down. You leave work at the office and you experience the relaxation that comes with just watching your favorite TV show or listening to your favorite music or reading your favorite book.

Take this and extend it for an entire weekend. Take one weekend out of the month and schedule a pajama day, a day where you get up and you wear your pajamas all day. Watch movies all day, popping popcorn, eating pancakes, playing games with the family, the children, the pets, but you do not come out of the pajamas all day long. This can be a surprisingly relaxing and fun experience.

When you do any of these activities (or lack of activities!), at first you might feel guilty. You'll find yourself thinking that you should be out being a productive member of society. Let that feeling pass. After a couple of Sundays where you've given yourself time to just rest, you'll really come to appreciate the value of the pajama day, especially when Monday comes 'round and you're actually energized and ready to attack the week.

Rest is a time for recharging and regeneration and healing of the body. When you allow this to happen, you'll be surprised at the results. Especially when it comes to the next part of your Wellness Blueprint, your relationships with others.

10
CONNECTIONS AND
COMMUNICATIONS
NURTURING YOUR RELATIONSHIPS

BY NATURE, WE ARE SOCIAL CREATURES AND WE interact with people constantly through our words and through our actions. Communications reflect our feelings, thoughts, personality, and our belief systems. In addition to our work relationships, our intimate relationships and our own self-esteem are reflected in the way we communicate with others.

When I was in high school, my mother used to tell me that I needed to smile more. She said I always looked like I "had an attitude." I never understood (or believed) her until I was chemistry class one day and a good friend of mine asked me, "Why do you always look mad?" It's funny how when your parents tell you something ,you never believe it; but when your friends tell you, you're quick to take a look at yourself. It's all about that need to fit in, that need for connection.

The way we communicate frames our connections with others. Connection with others—otherwise and hereafter known as *intimacy*—is defined as a closeness or a familiarity with another person. Intimacy comes about from reciprocal trust and safety between two individuals or between an individual and an entity. Intimacy comes in many forms and can be developed in many ways. That's what this part of the Wellness Blueprint is about. So, let's get a little bit closer.

BUILDING INTIMACY

Intimate relationships involve multiple aspects of sharing that evolve over time as a relationship becomes safely established. Intimate relationships are an integral part of overall wellness. As human beings, we are meant to interact with each other.

Given that we interact with many different types and roles of people every day, we should develop different types of close relationships. Such is the case with categories of intimacy. Closeness is fostered in different ways and for different reasons. The following table displays different types of intimacy.

TYPES OF INTIMACY	
Emotional	*Being emotionally vulnerable with another person.*
Intellectual	*Achieving closeness through the sharing of ideas.*
Sexual	*The sharing of erotic or physical closeness.*
Creative	*Closeness-involving creation together.*

TYPES OF INTIMACY	
Recreational	*Closeness related to sports, fun, and play of all kinds.*
Communicative	*The source of many of the aforementioned types of intimacy involving both verbal and non-verbal communication.*
Crisis	*A closeness that involves dealing with a struggle, loss, or pain.*
Conflict	*Closeness related to unity in argument or disagreement. Sometimes being in constant conflict with another creates an ironic intimacy, also known as co-dependency.*
Spiritual	*Closeness related to ideas of a higher power, shared belief systems, or the exchanges of a higher consciousness.*

Take a moment to reflect on these different aspects of intimacy. Can you think of connections that you have in different roles and with different people in your life that involve these different areas?

The brain is a social organ—we are literally hard-wired

for relationships and to be social. Research has shown that there is a kind of integration in close relationships that is health-enhancing. It has been also shown through research that *not* having nurturing interaction with others can be detrimental to a person's well-being. For example, children who are neglected emotionally or physically can be negatively impacted (become ill and even die[1]) from lack of connection. Studies have shown that newborns that are deprived of nurturing contact for long periods of time are at increased risk for Sudden Infant Death Syndrome (SIDS)[2]. Also, children who are emotionally neglected are more likely to suffer from depression, anxiety, social conduct disorders, eating disorders, and other mental illnesses. They are also more likely to take up attention-seeking behaviors such as promiscuity, fighting in schools, or even over-achievement, because they will do anything to be noticed whether the reinforcement is negative or positive.

One's intimate connections with others and one's emotional and psychological well-being has been shown to positively influence depression, heart disease, inflammatory bowel disease, and various forms of cancer. Fostering healthy intimate connections has even been shown to increase and improve the immune system and have a positive effect on reproductive health.

---

1 While it is obvious how the children who are physically neglected—not given food or water or left in unclean environments—would become ill, children who are emotionally neglected experience illness just as severe.
2 SIDS, also known as "cot death" or "crib death," is the unexplained death, usually during sleep, of a seemingly healthy baby.

THE FOUNDATION OF RELATIONSHIPS

So how can you foster healthy intimate relationships? Marriage researcher John Gottman studied thousands of couples over the last thirty years. In his book *The Seven Principles for Making Marriage Work*, he showed that the secret to a solid relationship is to build a friendship.[3] This involves cultivating some relatively simple skills and behaviors.

Δ   Building rather than fixing.

Δ   Being aware of others' attempts at making bids for connection.

Δ   Being aware of your responses to other peoples' bids for connection.

Δ   Being aware of "fuzzy bidding."

Δ   Respecting other peoples' boundaries and being clear about your own boundaries.

Build rather than fix. Building a solid foundation of friendship is one of the most important parts of building a lasting relationship. Friendship is born of fondness, admiration, and mutual respect. If our communication displays these characteristics, then even in conflict the relationship can still thrive. Dr. Gottman identifies what he calls "the four horsemen of the apocalypse," any of which, if permanently displayed in a relationship[4], predicts potentially fatal difficulties for that relationship.

Criticism	*Contempt*
Defensiveness	*Stonewalling (or ignoring)*

A major component of the "build rather than fix"

---

3   While Dr. Gottman's book is based on research of married couples, his results can be applied to other close relationships as well.

4   If they're displayed intermittently, it is not as much of a problem.

principle is appreciating the other person. It's important to appreciate the people that you're around. This applies to people at work, friends, and loved ones. It doesn't mean that you have to accept unacceptable behavior or become a doormat because you are just trying to be grateful for them; rather, it means appreciating the positive things about your loved ones, your colleagues, and your friends so that you can help balance the scales a bit when things are stressful. It also doesn't mean that you never get angry or upset with the people that you're around; rather you will appreciate them and accept them regardless of whether or not you're in disagreement. Remember the attitude of gratitude?

Try this exercise: Make a list of ten things that you appreciate about your companion or loved one.[5] Each day, let him or her know one or two of these things. Share the other things with someone else, perhaps in your loved one's presence. Add one or two things to that list daily. Notice how this affects your sense of closeness and appreciation for one another.

The idea of appreciating others is not exclusive to your significant other. In the realm of nurturing connection with the people in your life, this applies to your friendships, colleagues, work relationships, and family relationships. We often think about getting along and building relationships with those we consider very close to us. But how many times have you needed support at work or in the community? Do you think it's important to show the

---

5 If you currently don't have a companion or significant other, then use a close friend or relative.

same support and appreciation to those people that you might want from them?

Here is another exercise: Make a list of five things that you appreciate about your boss or employee and five things that you appreciate about your colleague or friend. Each day over the next week, give a show of appreciation to those people you put on the list. You will notice that while it puts a smile on their face, you will be the one with the warm and fuzzy feeling. More importantly, notice how this begins to affect your sense of closeness and appreciation for the other people.

Bids for Connection. When other people attempt to create connection through certain words or actions, it is called a bid for connection. They may be overt or subtle. An overt bid may be a direct request for time together. Some of the most significant bids, however, are the most subtle: making a joke; a subtle glance; a light pat on the shoulder; and, in this age of technology, a simple text message.

There are two basic kinds of bids: verbal and non-verbal. Verbal bids include thoughts, feelings, observations, opinions, and invitations. An example of a verbal bid may be a direct request for affection or to spend time together. Non-verbal bids for connection would be things like touching, facial expressions, a glance, affiliating gestures like a motion with the arm, or the OK sign or a thumbs-up, and vocalizing like laughter, grunting, or sighing.

Being aware of others' attempt to make a meaningful connection and responding is another way to foster closeness in an intimate relationship. Dr. Gottman opened what he has identified as the Love Lab at the University of Washington in 1990 to study numerous couples, looking at intimacy between them. While he initially thought that self-disclosure was the key to intimacy, what he found in his studies was quite different. In studying the couples, he found that it was the simple, daily interactions that most don't even think about that promote intimacy. Examples range from direct request for some quality time to the slightest glance or touch. These were the bids for connection that we just talked about.

Dr. Gottman found that there were three essential responses to these bids for connection: turning toward, turning away, and turning against.

Turning toward, in which the receiver of the bid responds positively to the bid with humor, respect, attention, affection, or a sense of joining. This response builds trust and respect and good feelings for the relationship over time.

Bid: *"Wow, there's a huge boat on the river."*
Response: "Is the river deep enough for it?"

Bid: *"This stupid computer. I am so sick of this job."*
Response: "Sounds like you need a break. Go get a cup of coffee and I'll find that number for tech support.

Bid: *"I can't believe that you were so late!"*
Response: "I'm sorry. I get that you're mad. Do you want to talk about it?"

Bid: "I don't suppose you'd ever think of going for a walk with me?"

Response: "I might. Hey, I've got an idea, do you want to go for a walk?"

These responses let the bidder know that they are being welcomed, understood, or joined. There is either an explicit or implicit communication that the bidder matters.

Turning away, in which the receiver ignores the bid by acting preoccupied. If this is a regular response, it can be very destructive to a relationship. There are three types of turning away responses:

Preoccupied response. The receiver is involved with another activity. For example, she wants to share her day and he wants to watch the news, so he ignores what she's saying.

Disregarding response. When the receiver ignores the bidder or focuses on insignificant details of the bid. For example, he tells her about a new car he wants to buy and she rambles about what color it should be, completely derailing his excitement.

Interrupting response. The receiver introduces unrelated matters or counter bids. For example, she tells him about a fear she's grappling with and he interrupts by talking about a new project he's beginning.

Do any of these responses sound familiar to you? Have you found yourself turning away from a bid for connection? Be aware as this can be very destructive to a relationship.

Turning against, in which the receiver of the bid responds in a manner that is belligerent, argumentative, hostile, or even filled with ridicule. This is also a very destructive behavior as it conveys disrespect and often contempt, which we identified earlier as one of the "four horsemen of the apocalypse."

Relationships are not likely to last as long with responses such as turning against. The five types of turning against responses are

Contemptuous   *Belligerent*   *Contradictory*
Domineering   *Critical*   *Defensiveness*

Contemptuous response. This is when the receiver responds with a hurtful, disrespecting comment or put-down.

Bid: "I think I lost some weight."
Response: "You, lose weight? I doubt it."

Belligerent response. The receiver is provocative or combative, as if they are looking for a fight. I bet we all have experienced a belligerent response and it does not feel good.

Bid: "You look tired, dear."
Response: "I wouldn't be if you helped me once in a while."

Contradictory response. The receiver seems ready for a debate or argument. It's less hostile than the contemptuous and belligerent responses, but it still blocks the attempt to connect.

Bid: "I just got a book about homeopathy and I'm excited to read it."
Response: "My friend says that stuff is just a bunch of voodoo."

Domineering response. The receiver attempts to control the bidder by getting them to withdraw, retreat, or submit. There is often a negative, parental tone. Have you ever found yourself being condescending to a co-worker, friend, or significant other?

Bid: "I just had a really tough day."
Response: "Now dear, that really is no way to behave. Why don't you go to your room until you've cooled off."

Critical response. The receiver issues a broad-based attack on the bidder's character using global terms like "always" or "never" or statements of blame or betrayal.

Bid: "I wish we'd talk more."
Response: "The problem with you is that you always let people down. You can never get anything right!"

Defensive response. This is where the receiver creates a sense of separation by disavowing all responsibility and being an innocent victim, thus discounting the reality of the bidder.

Bid: "I think you could have handled that client better."
Response: "I don't care what you say, I didn't do anything wrong. You are imagining the whole thing."

Do you recognize any of these behaviors in yourself? It's important when bidding for connection or when responding to bids for connection to be aware of your behavior and response patterns. Do you recognize how your response may be affecting the other person in the interaction?

Fuzzy Bidding. When bidding for connection, be

clear about what you're communicating. When the bid is not clear to the receiver, it can be confusing and can, in turn, draw an unintended response. Unclear bids for connection are called "fuzzy bidding."

"We never do anything fun."

"Why can't you be more romantic?"

"Why do you always ignore me when I'm talking to you?"

These are actual bids for connection, but they are riddled with complaint, criticism, or lament. They make it difficult for the receiver to respond in a positive, turning toward manner. The turnings away and turning against responses that we talked about earlier are actually the most common type of fuzzy bidding.

Take some time to recognize your own fuzzy bidding and notice how your partner responds to it. Notice how his or her response changes when you make your request more direct rather than indirect and negative. Notice when you are receiving a fuzzy bid from your friend or loved one and attempt to turn toward instead of against or away. Gently reassure them that it is okay to make direct requests for whatever they are bidding for—time, affection, fun. Notice how the response changes and notice whether the next time your loved one bids for connection it is more direct or not.

Respecting Boundaries in Intimacy. In healthy relationships there must be a balance between integration and differentiation—integration being *interdependence* and differentiation being *independence*.

If the scales are tipped too heavily to integration, the

couple can become enmeshed, which ultimately leads to co-dependence. In this case, there is no recognition or respect for boundaries and the two can end up losing their own individuality in each other. This is not a healthy situation.

An example of imbalance on the side of integration may be a couple that does everything together, has all the same friends, and neither have individual hobbies that they each like to do without the other.

In the cases where the balance is too heavily tipped towards differentiation, the two partners are so focused on their individuality that intimacy can be discouraged altogether. In this case, boundaries are rigid (more like walls) and the couple ends up sharing the same space at the same time with little else than that. This is also not the most sustainable situation in a relationship.

An example of the imbalance on the side of differentiation is a couple where each partner has a separate life, share no friends or activities that they like together, and only come home and live in the same house.

When integration and differentiation are at its ideal balance, there is a respect for each other's individuality and privacy, and at the same time the couple can, when desired, come together in supportive interactions on a daily basis. This actually promotes intimacy and self-disclosure and makes for a more stable and lasting relationship in the long run.

An example of a healthy balance between integration and differentiation may be a couple who share a love for poetry and music; however, he likes to play poker and has a poker night with his friends every Wednesday night and she loves volleyball and is on a league volleyball team. He attends her games and she makes snacks when the guys come for poker. In this scenario, they each have their own interests, but they support each other in these interests and they even share interests in which they come together on a frequent basis to enjoy.

Having a good balance between integration and differentiation also means that you must be clear about your own boundaries in addition to respecting others' boundaries. If you are not aware of your own boundaries, it makes it difficult to respect others.

A healthy relationship includes respecting others' boundaries and being clear about your own as well as a balance between integration and differentiation. If the scales are tipped too heavily toward co-dependence, the couple becomes enmeshed in which there's no recognition and respect for boundaries and the two can end up losing their own individuality. This can happen in friendships, in work relationships, in mother-child or father-child relationships, or in spousal relationships.

In the case where the balance is tipped too heavily to independence, the two partners are so focused on their own individuality that intimacy can be discouraged altogether. In this case, boundaries become rigid walls and the two people interacting end up sharing the same space at the same time, but little else than that.

In either case, a sustained connection is next to impossible.

CONFLICT IN RELATIONSHIPS

No matter how healthy and happy a relationship is, there will always be some amount of conflict. Dr. John Gottman has dispelled some long-held myths about what makes a stable and happy intimate relationship. One such myth is if you fight a lot, then you won't be happy with your partner and your relationship won't last. While it seems to be a reasonable theory, research doesn't substantiate it. Another myth is that if you don't confront your problems with each other and work through them in a mutually satisfactory way, you won't have a happy marriage. Dr. Gottman found that couples who fight frequently and couples that avoid conflict can be as stable and happy in their relationships as those couples that confront issues and calmly talk things through.

The most important factor in predicting marital longevity and satisfaction was the ratio of positive interactions to negative ones. In general, if a couple enjoyed five positive interactions to every negative one (a ratio of 5:1), then the partners had the best chance of happiness together. We have to remember, however we relate to one another, we all get upset with our partners from time to time. Sometimes when we get upset with each other, it results in a very intense emotional state that psychologists call "flooding," which alters our physiological functioning and hampers our ability to think. The most immediate cue to this powerful experience is the heart rate—it can increase up to 30 beats per minute within the space of a single heartbeat. The muscles tense, causing labored or decreased breathing and, most importantly, the ability to think clearly is severely reduced because the thinking part of the brain literally gets put on hold and the emotional part of the brain takes over.[6]

Take a moment to think when you have experienced flooding. The last time you were in an intense conflict with a person close to you, do you remember how your body felt? Can you remember your heart rate speeding up, your breathing speeding up, your muscles becoming tense?

What can you do in your relationships before flooding occurs?

When you are both calm, talk with your partner about how it feels when you enter into the emotional flooding stage and ask him or her how it feels when they get flooded. See if, together, you can devise a signal that will indicate that you're starting to flood—maybe even a code word—and that you need to take a break to calm down. This will allow time for the electrical activity in the limbic area to lessen and the adrenaline surge to lessen before you reach that "cornered animal" protection state where nothing productive can occur. Research has found that it takes twenty to thirty minutes after a flooding experience for the brain to reconnect and the adrenaline levels in the body to drop; so, give yourself plenty of time to come back to balance before you resume your discussion.

For the women: Keep in mind that men are much slower to return to that calm state than women. They tend to

6 For survival reasons, a part of the limbic area of the brain, which controls emotions, has the ability to bypass the cortex, the thinking part of the brain. It was undoubtedly useful when we were living in the midst of wild animals, but it can be damaging to our relationships.

experience flooding in a more intense manner than women and are more easily overwhelmed by relationship conflict. Research has also shown that men tend to maintain their distress longer by recycling their negative thoughts.

For the men: If you continue mentally rehearsing what you are angry about, then your brain will remain disconnected and you won't be able to process all the information and make a sound decision about how to proceed. You need to change your emotional channel and get your brain connected again. Here are some channel changers that work:

△ Physical activity like exercise or hard work.

△ Something requiring total concentration, like a complex game, a TV show or movies.

△ Meditation.

△ Deep breathing exercises.

△ Calling and talking with a skillful friend or coach.

Use whatever works for you to soothe yourself into a calmer state of mind and body—and then support your partner in doing the same.

Gottman's research has also revealed that women are usually the initiators of discussions about relationships problems. He says that relationship discussions invariably end on the same note that they began. If the conversation begins harshly, then flooding is more likely to occur and the end result is likely to be some variation of the above scene. Be mindful of how you begin and you'll be more likely to have a productive ending.[7]

7 In Steve Harvey's book *Act Like a Lady, Think Like a Man*, he wrote about how women initiate many conversations with men with the dreaded words "We need to talk" and how this causes immediate anxiety in men. Upon hearing those words, a man's brain tends to shut down and become defensive

We're all human, so we will get into conflicts where flooding will occur. But what happens after that? What do you do after the flooding occurs?

After you've calmed down and have normalized brain function again, take stock of the situation and evaluate what you need to do to reestablish closeness. Dr. Gottman calls these "repair attempts" and the magic words "I'm sorry" often does wonders. Sometimes it's just a touch or a look or an unrelated subject.

Very often, both partners completely miss each other's repair attempts, which can cause a lot of undue mental and physical stress. Like a bid for connection, the repair attempt can come in a myriad of forms that can only be recognized if you're present and your brain is integrated enough to be able to notice it. The elements that are necessary for repair are the same as those necessary for connection.

Generously pay attention to and appreciate each other and build a friendship as the basis of your relationship. Remember, it's never too late for a repair attempt, and most often the repair can actually build a stronger connection. When you understand the power of repair, it can help you to lighten up, which makes for a lot more fun in your relationship, whatever your relating style is.

RESOLVING CONFLICTS

Nearly all conflicts involve underlying emotional issues and the stronger the feelings, the more difficult the

---

almost immediately. It's not just men, though: women have a similar reaction to those words.

resolution. To resolve conflicts, then, it's absolutely necessary to address the feelings of all parties. The probability of a mutually agreeable solution is increased in conflict when:

△ The parties are direct in communication.

△ When the parties are honestly communicating both the thoughts and the feelings.

△ There is a mutual respect of the needs and the feelings between both parties.

△ Neither party feels superior or more powerful.

△ Participation is voluntary and not forced, and when the goal of both parties is a win-win situation.

So here are some basic steps to dealing with disagreement and conflict.

Seek to understand. Validate each person's feelings and confirm a willingness to solve the problems. If you seek first to understand, you will then be understood. Seek to understand the cause of the feeling that the person expresses to you and confirm that understanding by paraphrasing. Then, at this point, you might be able to identify the underlying (and perhaps unmet) emotional need. Also, you might show empathy, understanding, and compassion. Showing empathy doesn't necessarily mean that you have to agree with them. It just means that you have to show compassion for how they're feeling. Finally, you must ask the powerful and positive question of what would help you to feel better.

Seeking to be understood. This is honestly sharing

your feelings and needs and confirming an accurate reception and understanding of what these are. Be sure that when you're sharing your feelings and your needs that you're using mostly "I" statements, not "you" statements. "I" statements give the understanding that you're taking responsibility for your feelings and your needs; "you" statements convey blaming.

Mutually generate options and resolutions. Brainstorm solutions without evaluation or judgment. Discuss each person's feelings about the alternatives and, finally, make the selection that maximizes positive feelings and minimizes negative ones.

Sometimes you have to agree to disagree. Studies show that more than 50% of conflicts never get resolved. While that sounds bad, most often it's not because it's *how* you deal with the conflict that's going to foster a healthy continuing relationships. If you agree to disagree, you've essential resolved the conflict for the moment. If it's a situation where a decision absolutely has to be made, then you can come back to the table and eventually create a compromise using the same steps aforementioned.

A couple of other hints about resolving conflicts are to resist the inclination to focus on the person's behavior at the expense of addressing the feelings behind the behavior.

Also, allow the least powerful person to lead in generating and evaluating options. This helps balance the power.

Remember, if you are flooding and continue to mentally rehearse what you're angry about, you won't be able to process all of the information and make a sound decision about how next to proceed. Sometimes, you just need to "chill out."

CONNECTED

Relationships are an integral part of your life. When you allow yourself to make stable and healthy relationships, you, in turn, become a stable and healthy individual.

You may have noticed an overriding factor that creates these healthy, intimate relationships: communication. You are either communicating yourself properly or you're interpreting correctly.

The next chapter will cover in more detail communications and will be another step in your blueprint to health and wellness.

11
SPEAKING AND LISTENING
POSSIBILITY CREATED THROUGH LANGUAGE

DID YOU KNOW THAT ONLY TEN PERCENT OF communication is verbal?

Think about how well you know a spouse, child, or best friend. Do you know when they are lying to you? Most of the time, of course you do! Is it because they say, "I'm telling you a lie"? Nope. It's because you know their body language—you know their "baseline" and you know what it looks like when they deviate from that.

While words account a lot for how our message comes across and are not to be discounted, people primarily see the congruency between our words and our body language, facial expressions, the way we make eye contact, and the tone of our voice. It is a sign of integrity when we are congruent in our different aspects of communication. Our congruency in communication is the thing we leave people with in the end.

How authentic are you in communicating your messages? In previous chapters we talked about internal dialogs and thinking processes. Now we are going to tackle communication with others, and how it may directly or indirectly affect the states of your relationships. Let's begin by asking (and answering) some questions.

Are you being truthful and compassionate in your communication with others?

At first, you might say to yourself, "Yes, I'm pretty honest most of the time (or all of the time)." Dig deeper, though, and ask these follow up questions:

Do you say yes when you really mean no?

Do you say that you're fine, when you're really not?

Do you take your emotions out on others?

These are just a few ways that we dishonestly communicate with others. When we don't communicate what we are truly feeling, it places undue stress on our physical and mental states of being. Under this type of stress, we cannot be the best that we can be for the partnership. Be aware that just because we may communicate dishonestly sometimes doesn't mean we are dishonest by nature. However, we must take responsibility for our behaviors and know that when we become congruent in our communication, we will feel much less stressed and be much more authentic with others.

Are you able to assert yourself in order to be heard and understood?

Being assertive means that you are able to express yourself in a way that clearly states what it is that you need in a non-aggressive manner. When you are not able to assert yourself, you often end up committing to things that you don't want to do, being overworked, being self-neglected, and, eventually, becoming resentful, and sometimes exploding and becoming aggressive to overcompensate. Being assertive relates intimately with being truthful about your feelings. Not being heard creates resentments and tensions that collect within the body causing anxiety, depression, migraine headaches, high blood pressure, insomnia, and many other conditions that has stress as a contributor.

Do you acknowledge and apologize for mistakes you may make rather than covering them up?

This question requires a bit of self-honesty, as ego and pride can get involved when admitting to having made a mistake. While many people find it a weakness to admit to their wrong-doings, the truth is that it reflects integrity and strength of character when a person can swallow their pride and apologize for their mistake. Acknowledging, admitting to, and then learning from our mistakes is what contributes to our personal growth as human beings.

That being said, there are consequences to your actions—and admitting a mistake may not have a happy ending. But in the end, you will know that you acted in the highest integrity.

On the other extreme, there are those who over-apologize, even for things that are not their fault or responsibility. As we reviewed in previous chapters, it is important to know what is your "stuff" and what is not. If you truly did no wrong, then there is no need to apologize or make amends. You are not responsible for other peoples' feelings, behaviors, actions; nor are your responsible for environmental catastrophes, global warming, traffic, or delayed airplane flights! You are responsible for your feelings, words, and actions. That's it.

Are you a good listener?

Listening is just as much a part of communication as verbalizing. It conveys the message to others that you care about what they are saying to you. We all too many times want to be heard but as soon as it is our turn to listen we are interrupting the person talking to us at every other word.

Try this exercise: Use *the three-second rule*. Next time you are face-to-face or talking on the phone with your partner, do not start to speak until you hear at least three seconds of silence when they have stopped talking. (Count to yourself: "One-one -thousand, two-one-thousand, three-one-thousand.") If they remain silent, *then* give your response. You might find that the conversation goes much smoother.

When you are listening to your partner talking to you, give them your full attention. Stop what you are doing. You might pick up a message you never would have received had you been multi-tasking. You'll also find that when your loved one notices you giving them your undivided attention, they will appreciate you more and be more likely to reciprocate.

Do you offer unsolicited advice?

Though the intention may be honorable, giving un-

11 △ SPEAKING AND LISTENING

solicited advice can do more harm than good. Sometimes people just need someone to vent to—they need to
be heard. The next time a friend or family member calls
needing to talk, ask them, "Do you need me to just listen
or are you seeking feedback?" The answer will clearly define your role in the interaction.

*Do you frequently make absolutes, generalizations,
labels, or judgments of others when communicating?*

When we make absolute statements, generalizations,
and judgments, we are stating that we are not open to the
possibility of other options. When we are seeing things in
black and white terms, we are demonstrating inflexibili-
ty. Listen to your dialogue. Notice how often you use the
words "always" or "never."

*Do you avoid playing manipulative or psychological
games when communicating?*

Manipulation and psychological games are a form of
control. People tend to use them when they are trying to
get their way or get-over on someone else. Other times,
people may use them without knowing because that is
what was modeled to them from childhood.

Either way, it is a damaging form of communication.
If you think that manipulating others makes you clever or
powerful, know that the opposite is true. Keeping clean,
clear communication without walls or games is the best
way to foster positive and open interaction with others.

*Do you gracefully give and receive compliments and
appreciations to and from others?*

Everyone needs a little encouragement now and then—including you. It's okay to receive compliments for something admirable about you; so do so gracefully. As well, don't be afraid to dish out the joy! You can never know how a simple compliment may turn your loved one's day around, make an unbearable day just a little better, or stop tears from falling.

Exercise: Give your sweetie one genuine compliment everyday for a week—and see how it makes *you* feel. Notice the your partner's response, too! How does he or she react to the love? How does it affect your interaction on a daily basis as a couple? You'll see and feel the difference.

Effective Communication and Your Well-Being

We tend to look only at ourselves when it comes to wellness and relationships; we don't always consider how interaction with others can affect our well-being.

Think about how ineffective communication has affected all of the areas of your life.

With whom have you ineffectively or effectively communicated?

Effective communication is when the message you intend authentically comes across in a powerful (not forceful) way creating a new possibility or a desired outcome.

How has your ineffective communication affected intimate and close relationships alone?

How do you feel when you know you're getting your point across effectively?

*How do you feel when you know you have communi-
cated in an ineffective manner?*

SAFE/UNSAFE PEOPLE

Learning to identify safe and unsafe people (read:
knowing who will empowering you as opposed to people
who may leave you disempowered or simply commiserate
with you) is one of the most important factors in fostering
open and authentic communication. The reason it's important to identify the difference between these two types
people is because true connection cannot be cultivated
with people who are disempowering you. These people
may not be aware of it, but they often leave you feeling
more drained than enlivened.

What does safety have to do with it? If you do not
feel safe communicating with a person, are you (or pos-
sibly the person you are speaking with) likely to be fully
self-expressed? The answer is no.

Another reason you may tend to feel safer with some
people more than others is that the people with whom
you tend to feel safer usually operate with a higher level of
integrity—their lives are working, therefore, they are in a
better position to empower you. When there is no integrity, life tends to not work as well. People who have a lack
of integrity typically are not feeling whole and complete
themselves—and they are then not in any position to empower you. In fact, these are the people for whom "misery
loves company." The point is when there is no integrity,
openness in communication between you and another
person is not very likely—if not downright impossible.

So how can you tell the difference between someone who will empower you versus someone who will likely leave you drained and disempowered? Studies have shown that people who are creating a clearing for safety listen to you. Not only do they listen, but they *hear* you. They may make eye contact, acknowledging that they're with you. They validate you. They're non-judgmental. And they're real with you. Safe people are also clear and they have their own appropriate and clear boundaries. They're direct, usually supportive, loyal, and authentic.

People who are not creating a clearing for safe communication tend to not listen to you or hear you. They tend to reject, interrupt, and even invalidate you when you show them your true self. Sometimes they can be shifty-eyed, not making eye contact. They tend to reject and invalidate the true you. They may be judgmental or insincere. Many times people who are not in the game called "creating safe space for communication" are unclear in their own communication. They may say something to you in a way that is contradictory and difficult to understand, sending mixed messages. People who interact in ways that feel shady are indirect, competitive, and can be directly or indirectly dishonest. They may justify not telling the truth by omission as just "leaving out unimportant details." With a person who is not a clearing for safe interaction, the relationship tends to feel contrived and inauthentic.

Just because a person is not a clearing for safe communication doesn't mean you avoid them altogether. What it means is that *you* might become the clearing for powerful interaction—if you are up to the challenge. If you have the awareness of who is and who is not willing to be in a safe space of communication with you, then you are better able to determine how to approach communication with that person in a way that is powerful yet authentic and compassionate.

Let's do an exercise. Here are some examples of people you may have experienced in your life. Read each person's description and determine if that person is a clearing for safe communication or not.

A mother-in-law has a tendency to use guilt to control.

A father puts a contingency on helping a child out of a certain situation.

A sister plays the mother against the other sister for attention.

A friend tends to listen without judgment and without trying to offer unsolicited advice.

A significant other doesn't try to tell you how you need to feel or handle a situation, but instead shares his or her experience, strength, and hope on a similar situation to give you some perspective.

A friend tells you that they don't like your significant other, whom they haven't met, based only on a few conversations.

A wife invalidates her husband when he expresses concern of her working so much that they hardly see each other and get very little quality time together.

Let's go over the answers.

The mother-in-law who is using guilt to control is definitely **not a clearing for safe communication**.

The father who puts contingency on helping the child out is definitely **not a clearing for safe communication**.

The sister playing the mother against the other sister is **not a clearing for safe communication**.

The friend who listens without judgment and does not offer unsolicited advice is definitely **a clearing for safe communication**.

The significant other that doesn't tell you how to feel but only shares experience strength and hope? They're **a clearing for safe communication**.

The friend that makes a judgment against your significant other based on a few conversations. That's **not a clearing for safe communication**.

The wife who invalidates the husband when he tells his concerns to her is **not a clearing for safe communication**.

"DON'T GO TO THE HARDWARE STORE FOR BREAD"

Knowing who is and is not a clearing for safe communication ensures that you know who to go to when you need to express your authentic self or when you need to be vulnerable or ask for healthy emotional support.

Take a look in the mirror now. Are you being a clearing for safe communication?

Ask yourself the following questions:

Are you clear when you communicate?

Do you state plainly what your needs and boundaries are?

Are you honest?

Do you sugar coat or omit any important information?

Are you thoughtful in bringing your message?

Compassionate communication is more effective than hostile, defensive, or condescending communication. Are you respectful?

Are you assertive rather than aggressive in your communication?

Is your communication concise?

Do you beat around the bush in order to get to the point?

Is your communication culturally appropriate and sensitive?

Do you avoid making culturally insensitive jokes?

Is the conversation almost always about you and your problems?

Are you present during the conversation or are you "multi-tasking"?

Do you pause to listen during your communication?

If you're trying to attract people who are a clearing for authentic communication so that you can trust and build a connection with them, you must first become that which you desire. Take these questions to a close friend and ask them whether or not you do (or don't) do them. Far too often, we're oh-so-sure that we're doing all the right things, but we don't consider how other people perceive our actions and communication styles. You might even want to ask a few people that you trust, people with whom you feel safe to express your true self.[1]

If you noticed, most of the questions are yes or no answer questions. When you sit down with this person who is safe, explain to them that we don't need explanations of why or why not you are or are not communicating effectively in these different areas. Just ask them to answer yes or no. That's it. Then take your friend's answers, accept them for what they are, and work on what you need to.

TIPS FOR EFFECTIVE COMMUNICATION

Now that we've talked about what effective and ineffective communication is, let's go over communication tips to help you communicate and respond more effectively in general. Remember, conflict is created in language.

Avoid generalizations or use of absolutes. Deal directly with the issue in real time by referring to the situation as it occurs to you. Consider that how you view the situation may not be how it is actually happening. Resist resorting to colloquial clichés when speaking and instead use language that describes your experience and your view of it.

Ineffective: *"All men are dogs."*

Effective: *"I feel frustrated that I am not being treat-*

---

1 This is not an "opportunity" for people to gripe at you, to recklessly criticize you, to punish you, or to judge you. Nor is it a time for you to allow that. This is simply a way for you to inventory yourself. That's why it's very important to identify safe people with whom to do this exercise.

ed with respect by men like I deserve to be"

Avoid intimidation or condescension. Be compassionate and empathetic in your communication. Listening will give you a more powerful clearing to be heard than intimidation or condescension.

Ineffective: *"You feel ashamed? Well, that's ridiculous."*

Effective: *"You feel ashamed? I get that. Tell me why."*

Avoid labeling or judging. Be open to the view of the other person. Consider that just like what you do makes perfect sense to you within the construct of your view of the world, what they are doing also makes perfect sense to them within their construct of the world.

Ineffective: *"It's selfish of you for you to feel that way."*

Effective: *"Help me to understand what makes you feel this way."*

Avoid manipulation and ridicule. Be direct and open with your feelings. Manipulation and ridicule may have worked in the past to gain you the upper-hand, but it is guaranteed to eventually leave you alienated and, ultimately, unfulfilled.

Ineffective: *"Fine, don't come over. I'll just go find someone else to go out with."*

Effective: *"I was really looking forward to our time together. When can we reschedule that time?"*

Avoid blame. Take responsibility for your actions within the situation. Taking responsibility is different from assigning fault. Taking responsibility gives you the power to create a different possibility. It also gives the other person space to accept responsibility as well as a chance to co-create that new possibility.

Ineffective: *"We never get to spend time together because you are always working?"*

Effective: *"I know that I have not appreciated that you work hard to provide for us. How can we be creative in making quality time for each other over the next six months?"*

Avoid monopolizing conversations. Listen without expectation. Be present with the person you are listening to. You will find it a much more gratifying experience than being in a one-sided conversation.

Avoid communicating when emotionally flooded. Take a time-out to cool down. Then making a point to schedule a conversation to complete whatever needs to be resolved. When you are emotionally flooded, you are ruled by chemicals in the body that manifest as jumbled feelings and inarticulate (and often hurtful) words. Communication is hardly ever productive during this time because you are not in control, your machine is.

T.H.I.N.K.

There's an acronym that I like to use: THINK. It relates to the tried and true adage "think before you speak."

T-houghtful

H-onest

I-ntelligent

N-ecessary

K-ind

Keep those in mind when you are communicating with someone.

LISTENING TIPS

Listening is a very important and understated part of communication. Here are tips to improve your listening—and, therefore, your communication overall.

When you're listening to people, make eye contact. Actively listen. Head nods, gestures, and smiling convey to the person with whom your speaking that you're with them and listening.

Acknowledge the speaker. Be open to what the speaker is saying. Let the speaker finish their sentences or thoughts and avoid distractions like doing something else while they're talking. Multi-tasking while listening is one of the biggest ways to indicate that you don't care about what he person is saying. Don't interrupt, correct, or advise while you're listening. Likewise, don't spend time in your head preparing your response, otherwise you'll completely miss what they're saying.

Don't look away or walk away from a person when they're speaking to you.

Don't make disrespectful facial or body gestures, like eye-rolling or sighing or shaking your head negatively. This conveys judgment, contempt, and disapproval and it undermines the effectiveness of listening and communication overall.

COMMUNICATING FOR WELLNESS

Communicating—both the speaking part and the listening part—is one of the most important segments of your wellness blueprint. As you've been seeing throughout this book, one thing builds upon the other. Your communication habits forge your relationships; your relationships, in turn, come to comprise your environment. All of these together impact your overall wellbeing, either negatively or positively.

With how you communicate, you control a significant portion of this aspect of your wellness because it is you who is in command at all times.

Yes, all times. Even if a person who doesn't communicate well gets "in your face," you still have the choice of how to deal with that person. In that case, you could either devolve into arguing and allowing your flooded emotions to take control; or, you can respond calmly and collectedly, even disengaging for a few moments to collect yourself. The former will most likely lead to problems of all sorts. The latter will most definitely lead to well-being.

As you build your health and wellness, you will find that your communication habits will be the screws and nails that hold things together.

PART IV

PATHWAYS

If God can work through me, he can work through anyone.

—**St. Francis of Assisi**

12
EMOTIONAL INTELLIGENCE
BALANCE, AWARENESS, RESPONSIBILITY, AND EMPATHY

IN THE LAST FEW CHAPTERS WE'VE TALKED ABOUT dealing with our feelings, our thoughts, our emotions, communicating, and intimate relationships. In all of this, we're developing an **emotional intelligence**, which is your **emotional awareness** (knowing how you feel) plus your **emotional literacy** (your ability to express your feelings using "feeling words" in a three-word sentence, such as "I feel happy").

EMOTIONAL AWARENESS

There are several components to emotional awareness. **Acknowledging** is the first healthy step in the process of emotional awareness. You recognize that a feeling is present and you acknowledge the feeling. You may not be able to put your finger on it specific enough to verbalize it, but you acknowledge that there is some process in place.

Next is **identifying** the feeling. You label what you're feeling using feeling words, which range from vague to specific in meaning. To help you, here are lists of feeling words: positive, neutral, and negative.

POSITIVE FEELING WORDS

understanding	great	playful	calm
confident	courageous	peaceful	reliable
joyous	energeticat	ease	easy
lucky	liberated	comfortable	amazed
fortunate	optimistic	pleased	free
delighted	provocative	encouraged	
sympathetic	overjoyed	impulsive	clever
interested	gleeful	free surprised	
loving	concerned	eager impulsive	
considerate	affected	keen	free
affectionate	fascinated	earnest	sure
sensitive	intrigued	intent	certain

NEUTRAL FEELING WORDS

lazybored	lethargic	hopeless	tired
obsessed	greedy	rebellious	lonely
confused	longing	indifferent	
preoccupied	anxious	defiant	envious
emotionless	sleepy weak	surprised	
intimidated	thirsty cautious		thoughtful
boredom	respect apathy		cautiousness
avoidance	embarrassment	anticipation	
disoriented	indecision		

NEGATIVE FEELING WORDS

irritated	lousy	upset	incapable	enraged
disappointed		doubtful	alone	hostile

174

discouraged	uncertain	paralyzed	
insulting	ashamed	indecisive	fatigued
sore	powerless	perplexed	useless
annoyed	diminished	embarrassed	inferior
insensitive	fearful	crushed	tearful
dull	terrified	tormented	
sorrowful	nonchalant	suspicious	deprived
anxious	pained	grief	reserved
alarmed	tortured a	agitation	
apprehension	abandoned		

Now, write a couple of three-word sentences using feeling words. For example,

I feel excited.   *I feel distracted.*
I feel tired.   *I feel anxious.*

You get the picture. This is the foundation to recognizing and identifying your feelings on a regular basis.

Once you've identified the feeling, the next step is to **accept the feeling**. When you accept your feelings, you can then focus your energy on solutions and productive thoughts and actions.

After you've identified and accepted the feeling, the next step is to **reflect on the feeling**. The sooner you can accurately identify the feeling and reflect on it, the sooner you can take actions that are in your best interest to resolve whatever feeling it is.

Finally, we **forecast our feelings**. The ability to forecast your feelings gives you foresight to potential consequences of situations or for your choices and actions. This helps you to set appropriate boundaries. For example, if you know that you get irritable and unreasonable when you don't eat for extended periods of time, then you'll be sure to keep a snack with you at all times.

EXAMPLE: FORECASTING FOR HEALTH & WELLNESS

Here is an example of how forecasting has helped me avoid physical illness and emotional strain. When I was young, my mother loved to take us shopping. At first I would love to go because it meant getting new clothes or new shoes; but one of the downfalls of going to the mall with my family was that my mom could go and go and go and go—and never stop to eat a meal. I, on the other hand, have always been a girl who needs a regular meal. To this day, I eat something every few hours. If I don't, I get grumpy, have migraines, and, in general, get sick.

As I got older, I began to realize that whenever we went to the mall there were going to be prolonged periods of "starvation." I hesitated whenever my mother would ask if I would like to go shopping. I'd say no, then she would entice me with promises of new clothes. (And who can turn that down?) I'd give in, go to the mall, and have the same negative experience of being hungry and miserable because the family would shop for hours, dragging a hungry and tired me along with them.

One day, my mother asked me to go shopping. I paused before I answered to weigh the benefits and consequences: I was able to forecast that I would probably be miserable after about seven hours of shopping and no food. I finally said no. I set the boundary that I needed to in order to take care of myself. This was in no way an insult to my family; it was just a matter of me knowing what it was going to be like for them to be with a grumpy and irritable me because I couldn't eat. So I chose to stay home.

EMOTIONAL LITERACY

Developing emotional literacy is the process of expressing feelings using feeling words. You've already done a couple of feeling word exercises, but I want you to take a moment to write down ten positive feeling words and ten negative feeling words, without looking at the feeling words chart.

How is your feeling words vocabulary?

Our next step is to learn to express the intensity of our feelings. So, if you're saying ,"I feel tired," describe the intensity of the tiredness. Are you "extremely tired"? "slightly tired"?

Think about what you're feeling now. Can you put a level of intensity to your feeling?

Another component of emotional literacy is using "I" instead of "you" messages. We talked about this in communication. "I feel…" versus "you make me feel…" is an indicator of emotional literacy. Think of examples when you have used "I feel…" instead of "you make me feel…."

Next, avoid indirect communication of your feelings. This is probably one of the most common things that people who are learning emotional literacy do: they use "I feel like…" instead of "I feel…." For example,

Indirect: "I feel like you are rejecting me."

Direct: "I feel rejected."

Indirect: "I feel like you are not listening to me."
Direct: "I feel ignored."

With indirect communication, you need to make sure you have an awareness of your non-verbal communication. 90% of all communication is non-verbal. As you develop your emotional literacy and your emotional intelligence, you become very good at reading non-verbal cues in communicating. With practice, you will integrate these tools and your overall emotional intelligence will strengthen, which will, in turn, improve your communication with others and your relationships overall.

EMOTIONAL HONESTY

Along with being emotionally aware and emotionally literate, you must be honest in expressing your emotions. How many times have you disregarded your own feelings in order to make someone else happy? Can you remember a time where you have been asked how you felt and you "lied" to protect the other person's feelings or even to protect another person's perception of you?

When you are emotionally dishonest, you lose out on the true value that your real feelings have to offer. Not only are you being false, inauthentic, and insincere, your emotionally dishonesty creates a general mistrust in yourself, in your relationships, and even in society as a whole.

When you are honest with your emotions, you encourage similar openness and honesty in all of your relationships: your co-workers, friends, family, and everyone in between.

Emotional honesty requires more energy than denial of

our true feelings. It requires a level of awareness of our emotions first of all; we must also be self-confident and courageous to be able to express our true feelings at all times. It's easier to be dishonest emotionally because society encourages us to hide our true feelings or tell "little white lies" for the "greater good" sometimes. Even from an early age, we are taught to repress what we really feel.[1] As adults, when we try to be honest with our feelings, we are sometimes ridiculed, invalidated, ignored, and even attacked. This further discourages open expression of our feelings.

So, how do you foster emotional honesty in relationships? The primary way to create safe environment for emotional openness is through **emotional validation**. When you validate someone's feelings you are showing them that you accept their unique identity and individuality. In some ways, it's a practice of tolerance and, even more so, compassion.

The steps to emotional validation are:

△   Acknowledging the other person's feelings.

△   Identifying the feelings.

△   Active listening.

△   Helping the other person label the feelings.

△   Being present emotionally and physically for the person.

---

1   Children start out as relatively honest by nature. They freely express their true feelings and emotions. Then adults send them messages that encourage them to act in a way that is inconsistent with what they feel, such as asking them to smile even when they feel sad or telling them to apologize for things for which they feel no regret and even forcing them to say "thank you" for things for which they feel no appreciation. These early inconsistencies ingrain in their minds the basic principles of hiding and/or lying about how they really feel for the benefit of someone else.

△ Being patient.

△ Being accepting and non-judgmental.

THE B.A.R.E. NECESSITIES

To conclude this chapter of the Blueprint, I give you the **B.A.R.E Necessities of Emotional Intelligence**.

B-alance

A-wareness

R-esponsibility

E-mpathy

When you're balanced, you're free of cognitive distortion and impulse control, you allow delayed gratification, and you have a sense of emotional detachment when necessary.

When you're aware, you're able to acknowledge and identify specific feelings. You're also able to forecast feelings for certain situations.

With responsibility, you're taking responsibility for your own feelings—for your fears and desires and everything in between. You're taking responsibility for your own thoughts and beliefs, knowing what's yours and what's not yours. You're taking care of your feelings.

Finally, with empathy, you have awareness and acknowledgment of the other person's feelings and needs. There is a sensitivity, a compassion, an understanding for others.

Do you see how this is starting to integrate back into the other aspects of balance in life? The B.A.R.E. Necessities of Emotional Intelligence include self-responsibility; self-love; taking responsibility for your thoughts, actions, beliefs and feeling; communicating effectively so as to foster healthy relationships; and being sensitive and empathetic and compassionate towards others.

One final thought on emotional intelligence: you don't always have to understand why people do what they do or feel what they feel. We all have different life experiences, beliefs, expectations, and insights. The primary goal of improving your emotional intelligence is to better notice how those around you feel. By doing so, you can then make better choices—from how to communicate with a person to actions you will take.

Again, one step builds upon the ones before it. And each new tool you learn goes into your "tool chest," ready to be used whenever you need it.

13
MAKING IT MATTER
YOUR CONNECTION WITH A HIGHER SOURCE

I GREW UP IN A MEDICAL BACKGROUND: MY MOTH-
er is a holistic dentist and my father is an obstetrician/gy-
necologist. Thus, from the time that I was in grade school
I knew that I wanted to become a physician—a doctor.
Once I got into college, I began to learn more about esoter-
ic forms of healing like yoga therapy and massage therapy
and reiki therapy, all which have become more mainstream
but which were, at that time, considered somewhat "out
there" by most medical professionals. When I was in the
process of applying to medical schools, I began receiving
mail from alternative medical schools—schools of naturopathy, herbal medical programs, DO (Doctor of Osteop-
athy) programs. Even though those were tempting to me,
I had this sense—a feeling—that I needed to continue on
my path to the traditional schools to which I was applying.
That was not to say that I didn't have a strong interest in
the naturopathy schools, but I didn't quite know enough to
veer off the path that I was on.

When I was in medical school (Morehouse School of
Medicine), I discovered reiki energy healing. I felt intuitive-

ly called to it, so I trained in it. (I often chuckle about that today; I was actually a healer before I was a doctor.) After finishing medical school, I began to realize that my path was going to be different from my fellow doctors. I was very interested in traditional Chinese medicine. (I had even, ordered traditional Chinese medical texts and began to study them alongside of my traditional medical texts.) I was interested in all aspects of healing and how I could use them along side what I learned in medical school. So, when I applied to my residency in family medicine, I already had the awareness that when I finished, I would likely pursue some form of holistic training. However, I didn't know what it looked like, so I had to continue following the breadcrumbs that were being strategically placed by my Higher Power.

Over the next five years, paths became available to further my training and opportunities opened that led me to opening up my own wellness practice, Mind Body Spirit Wellness Inc. The most important part of this was that by not holding on to what I thought it needed to look like, I was able to fully realize my true calling. To this day, my path is evolving and changing daily. By trusting in the process—and doing the footwork—I am allowed my continued growth and success today.

It would have been easy for me to come out of my residency, get a regular job, and make plenty of money right away. Frankly, it was very tempting. That would have come at a huge cost: had I narrowed my true passion for healing for the sake of money, I would be completely miserable today. My creativity would have been stunted and I wouldn't have the blessing of being able to empower and educate people through the many mediums that I do to-day—all because I denied living authentically.

Living an authentic life helps you to find meaning; it helps you to find your passion. When you are totally connected with your authentic self, you are also connected to your higher source.

How do you find meaning in life? How do you connect with your authentic self? To find those answer, let's begin by taking an inventory.

WHERE ARE YOU NOW?

Where are you in your life now? Let's figure that out by doing a life audit spin. In this spin, you'll take the twelve dimensions of wellness and assess where they are now and then reflect on where you would like them to be.

My self-love is _____.

My self-responsibility is _____.

My breathing is _____.

How I eat is _____.

My movement is _____.

My senses are _____.

My feelings are _____.

The way I think is _____.

My work is _____.

My fun time is _____.

My relationships are _____.

How I find meaning in life is _____.

My relationships to my higher power is _____.

How satisfied are you with your answers? Would you like to see improvement in any of these dimensions? By now you already know what improvements you would like to make based on the previous chapters. Learning to live in your authentic self by connecting with your higher power is the bow that creates this beautiful gift that is *living life on your terms.*

A PLACE OF AUTHENTICITY

Are you acting from a place of authenticity? Answer these statements true or false.

I love what I do in my career.
I take time to do fun things that I like regularly.
I say what I mean and mean what I say, without saying it mean.
I know exactly who I am.

If you answered false to any of those statements, then you may not be living from your true to your authentic self. That means that you need to identify what it is in your life that keeps you from living authentically.

Here is a list of things that might be preventing or hindering you from living a life congruent with your authentic self.

Δ   Not loving your career or what you do in life.

Δ   People pleasing and other forms of "dishonest" communication rather than speaking and expressing yourself honestly.

Δ   Doing the things you don't want to do because that is what your partner or friend wants to do.

Δ   Not doing what you want to do because of someone else.

Δ   Not expressing your true emotions or not expressing emotions at all.

Δ   Not taking time for fun and relaxation.

Δ   Not being in touch with your inner child.

All of these are examples that can keep you out of your true self. Let's take one of these examples and do a spin on the Wheel of Wellness using the statement,.

When I am not in my authentic self, my (dimension) is _____.

Do this exercise with all the dimensions.

self-love   breathing   eating   moving
sensing   feeling   thinking   working
playing   intimate relationships
your ability to find meaning in life
your relationship to your higher power

Once you have looked at the consequences of not living in your authentic self, look at the benefits of living in your true self. Use the reverse of the statement above and do the same spin around the Wheel, this time using,

When I am in my authentic self, my (dimension) is

_____.

FLOW EXPERIENCES

In the process of living authentically, we acknowledge our intuitive self—our higher self. When we are accessing that higher self, we experience more **flow** in our lives. What is flow?

Some call them coincidences or synchronistic events or divine interventions or intuitive experiences. I like to call these experiences *divine experiences*.

During the editing of this book, my practice began to experience exponential growth—so much so that I began to think I needed to add a new physician to my practice. I wasn't completely sure of how or where I was going to find this doctor, but I simply declared that it was time to expand and asked God to provide me with the right person. About a month later a young physician whom I had mentored years ago walked into the office to see me for coaching. She told me that she was ready for a career change and that she wanted to focus more on wellness and holistic care. I could hardly contain myself! In fact, I didn't even try to hold back. I asked her if she would be interested in joining my practice. She was ecstatic. Shortly afterwards, I became pregnant. My due date coincided perfectly with her projected starting date. She has since joined the practice and is fitting in perfectly. This was perfect flow at it's best.

However, that is *not* the end of the story. Soon after she joined, we began to experience a high demand for weekend hours, which neither myself nor our new doctor covered. After a short deliberation, I decided I'd find a Physician's Assistant to cover Saturdays. The only caveat was that he or she would have to already have the experience in all of the integrative therapies I already provide—and that is not very common my area. Nevertheless, I began my search and within one week, I found not one but *two* perfect fits who were willing to work alternate Saturdays so that all Saturdays are covered! What are the chances that this would happen so fast? Slim! Perfect Flow!

This is just one example of the flow experiences that I have experienced—and have created. (Yes, created!) My intention, combined with integrity and action, produced an amazing result.

The key to flow experiences is recognizing the synchronistic events that usually come with them. For example, calling someone who states that they were just thinking about you; following your intuition on a particular decision that leads you to more open doors; listening to a bad feeling and avoiding a catastrophe.

And remember integrity: Living your life by honoring your word is what makes your life work. It's what makes these flow experiences manifest abundantly.

Think about your past week. What seemingly coincidental things have happened in your life? Write them down. Share them with someone else. Bring yourself to the awareness of these events as flow experiences. You'll begin to recognize these synchronistic events more often.

Being in the present moment[1] is essential to recognizing these flow experiences or synchronistic experiences. What are some ways that you can be present in life today?

1 There's an old proverb that I love: "The past is gone and the future is not here yet, but what we have today is a gift and that's why God calls it the present."

Let's do another spin on the Wheel of Wellness.

When I am present in the moment, my self-love and self-responsibility are _____.

My breathing is _____.

My eating is _____.

My sensing is _____.

My feeling is _____.

My moving is _____.

My thinking is _____.

My working is _____.

My playing is _____.

My intimate or close relationships are _____.

My ability to find meaning in life is _____.

My connection with my higher power is _____.

Reflect on how the dimensions of your life are affected when you are right in the present moment.

LIVING IN THE PRESENT MOMENT

Try this exercise: Have a conscious and mindful day. Wake up and set the intention that everything you do that day will be from your intuitive self. Let every decision you make come from pure intuition and gut—not logic or straight emotion. As they say, follow your "first mind" that day.

Let's revisit some tools that we mentioned earlier that can help you to be in the present moment and to get in touch with your authentic self.

Affirmations. Remember that an affirmation is a positive statement in the present tense that affirms a particular goal or desire, such as "I love and accept myself unconditionally" or "God gives me all that I need, all of the time." Create your affirmations, and say them frequently.

Visualization. Remember that visualization is creating a mental image in your mind of a particular action or intention. It's used in many forms by athletes and business people, and even in meditation and progressive relaxation. We did a visualization earlier in the book for relaxation purposes; now use visualization to create the intention of being in touch with your higher consciousness.

Gratitude. Gratitude has come up several times in this book. How does it create flow? Focusing on what you are grateful for brings you right into the present moment. It shifts your thinking from negative to positive. In doing so, it connects you with your higher power. It creates an open channel to receiving more abundance. Earlier in the book one of the exercises was to begin doing a gratitude list on a daily basis. Adding to this exercise, you can create a gratitude list even on the things that haven't happened yet. It's called "*thanking* as if," a concept similar to "acting as if." You can speak of gratitude for your intentions, gratitude for the things that you desire, and, of course, gratitude for the things that have happened or the flow experiences that have come.

While these tools may not be new, keep in mind that we're not here to reinvent the wheel. What we are doing is reminding you of all the tools you have readily available around you in your everyday life. You have tools that can—and will—bring you closer to living the life that you want, if you utilize them.

GETTING IN TOUCH

What are other ways of getting in touch with who you really are?[2]

- △ Journaling
- △ Making a list of your likes and dislikes
- △ Spending quality time with yourself
- △ Listening to your intuition

You can do any or all of these things. What is most important is that you find the things that work for you.[3] Ask yourself what of these things helps you to connect with your higher power. Whether or not you are religious, connecting to a power greater than yourself can help you begin to connect with your authentic self.

If you're a person that is not sure that you believe that there is a power greater than yourself, that's okay. Think about the things in your life that you have needed help with that seemed to miraculously sort themselves out. Think of something that was out of your control that you just had to completely surrender. Recognize those times when you

---

2 Some of you out there are saying, "I already know who I am." That's great! But even if you do feel like you know who you are, these are some great exercises that will help you to continue to be in touch with yourself.

3 Poetry, yoga, dancing, and spiritual fellowship help me connect with my higher consciousness and my higher power, which make it easier for me to listen to my intuition on a daily basis.

had done all you could for a situation and as soon as you let it go it worked out by itself. This acknowledgment is a start in identifying a power greater than yourself.

For those of you who believe that there is a power greater than yourself, but aren't too sure what it looks like, I want to introduce you to an exercise that will help you begin to formulate that connection. This is also great if you want to explore and deepen your established relationship.

Write a description of what your higher power would look like if you could see Him, Her, or It. Describe the colors, smells, and the feeling you get when you are connected to that being. What do you call it? Where do you connect best? How do you connect best? Do you feel surrounded by that power in nature? With music? How do you communicate with it? Do you communicate as though you're talking with your best friend? Through prayer, meditation, yoga? Just take a moment and reflect and write about how you most feel connected to the universe.

Next, write a job description for the God or Higher Power of your understanding. Write all of the characteristics and requirements that you would like for your higher power to have. Then reflect. Does your current concept of a higher power fit this job description? If not, then would you like for it to? How will you begin to shift your perception to make your ideal higher power congruent with your current higher power?

Another block of communication with our higher source tends to be how we think our higher power sees us. I recently had a client and when we did work around her higher power, it was revealed that, while she had grown up in a Christian church, her perception of what her higher power thought about her was that He was judging her for not having gone to church every Sunday and for becoming a little bit estranged (or what she thought was estranged) from her connection with Him. In doing a little bit more work with her, I asked her to write a letter from the eyes of her God to herself and to use the concept of her ideal higher power to write this letter and not the concept of her old higher power. She wrote that her god loved, forgave, accepted, and was non-judgmental to her. With more work around that idea, I asked her why her higher power couldn't be just like the one that she wrote about in her letter. This was a major breakthrough for her. She began to realize that she could form her own personal relationship with the higher power and that it does not have to be judgmental or punishing. He can be a loving and accepting higher power with whom she could connect in whatever way was most comfortable for her.

Acknowledging your core—as we've talked about throughout this book—is about being honest with yourself and how you are feeling. To acknowledge your thoughts and feelings is to acknowledge who you truly are and honor that person.[4] You don't have to react or do anything; just be mindful of yourself. Know that self-love and self-acceptance comes wherever you are. We are all human and life is a process. Remember the quote from Shakespeare: "To thine own self be true." If you're not taking care of yourself, you will not be effective for anyone else.

4 This is also a practice in emotional intelligence, a concept mentioned earlier.

When you are true to yourself, you are living with congruency, your inside thoughts and feelings match your outside actions. You say no when you mean no and say yes when you mean yes.[5]

This last step—living in your true authentic self and acknowledging and nurturing your relationship with your higher source—connects to everything that we've already talked about. Repetition helps to set things in the permanent consciousness.[6]

Another way of connecting is service and random acts of kindness. We cannot talk about receiving without talking about giving. Get out and volunteer your time and your talents. Help others. It is said that in order to keep what you have, you must "give it away." These random acts of kindness do not have to be huge; they could be something as simple as complimenting a complete stranger or reaching out to connect with an old friend; acting on someone else's behalf without needing to be recognized.

Make a commitment to be of service. Start with once a quarter, then move to once a week, then once a month. What you will notice is not only how this makes others feel good, but how it makes you feel great. By performing these random acts of kindness you'll begin to have more flow experiences—more connection with that power greater than yourself—and you'll begin to find your inner authentic self and live in it on a daily basis.

Remember awareness, acceptance, and action. Be

5 You say what you mean and mean what you say without saying it mean.

6 This is how we integrate these lessons into our innermost cellular self. I want you to be able to put this book down and remember just every concept in it, and that is why themes are being repeated and intertwined for your benefit.

aware of synchronistic events and acknowledge them, even the small ones. Become aware of those experiences that you may have passed off as just coincidences. The more you acknowledge them, the more you will recognize when they come and more will appear.

Recognize the experiences as potentially more than just coincidences. Accept that there may be a higher purpose. At this point you don't need to do anything: accepting is just that—processing. As you recognize these flow experiences, they start to happen more frequently. In other words, you create more flow—and that's the action.

Remember the stories I told earlier. The more we recognize and acknowledge them as flow, the more they happen. I am co-creating with my higher power—and so are you.

Continue to take an inventory of your authenticity. At least once a month do a spin on the Wheel of Authenticity. You can do these at any time.

Finally, don't be put off by negative reinforcement. You will always encounter nay-sayers on your journey to being healthy and happy. Oftentimes, as you begin to reclaim yourself, others, who are used to you acting for them, will rebel at first. Remember that it's not about them. You are responsible for your own serenity—and your own health and wellness.

As a wise man[7] once said: "Be who you are and say how you feel. Those who matter won't mind, and those who mind don't matter."

7 Bernard M. Baruch.

14
BEYOND THE BLUEPRINT
WHERE DO YOU GO FROM HERE?

HOLISTIC MEDICINE IS A GROWING AND INCREAS-ingly demanded specialty today—and many doctors are beginning to jump on the bandwagon, adding "holistic" to their tag-lines in order to gain more appeal and meet the demands of patients. How do you know when you are getting a true holistic doctor versus a traditional doctor who is simply calling themselves "holistic"?

Here are a few things to look out for and a few questions to ask when searching for a holistic doctor for yourself and your family.

WHAT IS HOLISTIC MEDICINE?

To know whether you are finding what you are seeking, you must first know what you are looking for. The medical version of The Free Dictionary defines holistic care as

> *a system of comprehensive or total patient care that considers the physical, emotional, social, economic, and spiritual needs of the person; his or her response to illness; and the effect of the illness on the ability to meet self-care needs.*

This is distinct from the definition of Integrative

Medicine, which is

the "new medicine": a term for the incorporation of
alternative therapies into mainstream medical practice.

Not all integrative medicine practitioners are holistic in mindset or practice, nor are they mutually exclusive. The question to ask yourself is, *Do you want an integrative medicine doctor, a holistic doctor, or a combination of the two?*

WHAT IS THE DOCTOR'S TRAINING?

Like any physician, when you are looking for a holistic doctor, you want to know about their training. Is this a traditional physician that has done extra training in an integrative or holistic discipline such as acupuncture, coaching, homeopathy, naturopathy, or the like? Does this physician do regular continuing medical education specific to the holistic modalities that they incorporate?

Keep in mind that only in recent years have formal residencies and fellowships in integrative medicine been developed. There are many phenomenal holistic physicians who have years of experience in holistic practice who have not done these residencies. Most of these physicians may have begun their practice in other specialties, such as family medicine, internal medicine, pediatrics, or obstetrics/gynecology, and transitioned into holistic medicine.

Don't be afraid to ask your potential doctor about his or her training and background.

WHAT IS THE DOCTOR'S MISSION STATEMENT?

You can tell a lot about the physician(s) and how holistic they are by looking at their mission statement and their website. When you look at their website, do you get a sense of them being holistic in nature (even if they are integrative practitioners)?

To take this a step further, call the office and ask to speak with the physician to get a feel for that practitioner. If you have specific questions about their services, most holistic doctors are happy to call you and briefly speak with you to make sure you get your questions answered and have a sense of feeling valued as a potential patient.

WHAT ARE THE OFFERINGS OF THE DOCTOR AND THEIR PRACTICE?

Look at their website to get a feel for the types of services and products that the physician and practice offers that are considered holistic in nature. Does the physician perform holistic services themself or do they have a partnership with other holistic or integrative practitioners? Do they sell supplements? If so, is there pressure to purchase the supplements from them as opposed to them recommending supplements that you may get elsewhere?

Whatever the case, you just want to be sure that what they offer is congruent with what you are looking for.

You also want to be comfortable with the office practitioners, the doctor himself, and the staff.

DOES THE DOCTOR LIVE THE LIFESTYLE THEY TEACH?

This is very important. While we are all constantly working on improving and transforming certain aspects of our lives as holistic practitioners, it is important that the physician's actions and lifestyle are congruent with what they are teaching. While a physician who is not practicing what they "preach" may not affect their ability to treat their patients effectively, it certainly makes a difference in the credibility of the practitioner when you can see that they "practice what they preach." Furthermore, you as a client will feel more confident and empowered knowing that your holistic doctor sees the same value in his or her life in practicing those things that he or she is recommending to you.

These are a few simple things to look at when searching for a holistic doctor that is going to give you exactly what you need as a patient. Once you have found the physician, make sure you are left empowered, listened to and heard, and fully taken care of at the end of each visit and that all of your needs were addressed. A good holistic doctor literally leaves nothing on the table, even if it takes a little more time or more than one visit to get everything sorted out.

THE DOCTOR PATIENT RELATIONSHIP

Once you have found the doctor that is right for you, how do you foster the ideal doctor patient relationship?

There was a tome when a patient went to the doctor and the doctor did *all* the talking. The doctor asked the questions, made the recommendations, gave the prescriptions, and sent the patient on their way. But the information superhighway—known as the World Wide Web—has changed all of that. Now we have *WEBMD*, *Medscape*, and many other medically related and diagnosis information sites that allow the consumer (you) to educate themselves about their health and their condition.

Thus, the doctor patient relationship has changed and continues to evolve. It is important to know that even with the abundance of information out there on health and wellness, the doctor patient relationship is still a sacred relationship. When you go to the doctor, you are entrusting them with your health—and sometimes with some very personal things. There are still some very "old school" docs out there that believe that "what the doctor says goes."[1] If that works for you, the fine; run with it. If not, know that you have many options available to you, most of which are a mouse-click away.

PATIENT PARTICIPATION

It is important today for patients to participate in their health.[2] This means taking responsibility for their habits and roles in care. This may start in the doctor's office, but it goes on to everyday life.

I saw a patient who was very insistent that she had a thyroid problem because she couldn't lose weight (I can't count how many times I've heard that one). When I began to question her about her habits, she admitted to eating fast food almost daily, not exercising, and practicing a number of other unhealthy habits. This was a clear lack of insight—and, therefore, participation—on her part.

On the other hand, I saw a patient who thought she

1 At this point in the book, it should be obvious that I have a different opinion.
2 Again, at this point in the book, that should be quite obvious.

might need a referral to a podiatrist (foot doctor) because of chronic foot pain she had been experiencing for years. She gave me a very thorough history of her habits, of past evaluations (which were confirmed when I checked her chart), and a very specific description of where and when her pain took place. I evaluated her and determined that the localized pain in her foot was due to a plantar wart[3] that was causing pressure and pain in her foot. She asked me how she may have gotten it and I gave her several possibilities (walking bare-foot on the floor or shower, using some else's socks or slippers). She asked me about different options for treatment and I explained the different options including cryotherapy, over-the-counter wart removal, and surgical removal. I recommended cryotherapy as a start and she agreed. In this case, there was active exploration on both the doctor's and the patient's part, which lead to a more thorough evaluation and management decision.

DOCTOR EXPERTISE

It is very important to remember that although *Web-MD* and similar websites provide a wealth of information, they also provide a disclaimer that they are not to be substituted for a physician's evaluation. Far too often I have patients come to me who have already diagnosed themself and plotted their evaluation and treatment course. While I think the educated patient is refreshing (and I actually encourage patients to tell me what they've researched

---

3 Plantar warts are noncancerous growths caused by a virus (the human papillomavirus) when it enters the skin through small cuts or abrasions. While they are not a serious health threat and there are sundry self-treatments, sometimes a doctor is necessary to remove them.

and found), patients need to be aware that physicians went to medical school and residency and some of us fellowships—often totaling over twelve years of education, training, and experience.

Please let me be clear: if patients have questions about new treatment options or treatments they've heard about on TV, then they absolutely should ask. However, demanding a course of treatment because you—as the patient—think you know better because you read it on the Internet is highly inappropriate—and sometimes even offensive to some physicians. More than that, it can also be dangerous.

The bottom line is to just take caution on how you approach your physician with your research.

Fostering a good doctor-patient relationship goes both ways. A physician should not only be competent (obviously), he or she should also be open to allowing patients to participate in their care. A good physician will seek to educate the patient about management decisions and be open to any questions that arise.

A HEALTHY TOMORROW AND BEYOND

By now you should get the main idea of The Wellness Blueprint: your health and wellness is, ultimately, in your own hands. You can't expect to live a life of bad habits and activities and then visit a doctor when you feel sick and expect the doctor to give you a pill that will magically make it all go away. Life—and health and wellness—just doesn't work that way.

If you want to lose weight, sure there are plenty of

"pills" (both literal and figurative) that will make you thinner, everything from diet pills to liposuction. It's been shown all too often, though, that their efficacy is short-term while their affects on health can be destructive. The best option is to take responsibility, form good habits, and wage "the long war" rather than the "quick fix."

If you suffer from a chronic condition, then you'd be amazed at how making just some of the small changes recommended in this book can allow you to have a better—if not outright wonderful—quality of life. I've seen people who suffered from chronic pain who, while they will never be totally pain-free, live full and active lives because they began practicing yoga therapy.

Too many people, primarily those in the United States, think of themselves as a car and doctors as mechanics; and when something goes wrong, all they need to do is go to get things "fixed." Unfortunately, that's too often untrue.

Even more unfortunately (and continuing with the car-mechanic analogy), more people take better care of their cars than they do themselves: they perform routine and regular maintenance, they avoid driving on bad roads or in unsafe conditions, they wash and wax and polish. Yet for their bodies and their health and wellness, they do nothing of the sort: they eat whatever, they allow themselves to be lazy and sedentary, and they visit a doctor only when things reach a point where the discomfort is too much. And then they expect the "mechanic" to fix it and make it all better.

Your health is yours and yours alone. Yes, some people get the short-end of the stick due to genetics or environment or just plain bad luck. Yes, there are people who can inhale a box of donuts and not gain a pound, yet others will just look at the box and gain a pound. But each one of us makes-do with the hand we're dealt.

As is often said, "It is what it is."

I also frequently say something else: "Don't get it twisted." What I mean by that is even if you were dealt a really bad hand, that doesn't give you an excuse to give up and give in and wallow. Quite the contrary: it means that you just have to dig in, maybe work at things a little harder than most, and overcome what was dealt to you.

This book was written to be your starting point on your path to health and wellness. It's an opportunity for you to take and reclaim your health and wellness and make them your own. Seize it and run with it.

A person can have all the riches in the world. All the power in the world. Without health, it's all for nothing.

And it all begins with you.

References and Resources

Books

Cohen, S., Gottlieb, B.H., Underwood L. (2000). *Social relationships and health.*

Cohen, S., Underwood, L. & Gottlieb, B.H. (Eds). *Social support measurement and interventions: A guide for health and social scientists.* New York: Oxford University Press.

Gottman, John PhD. (1995). *Why marriages fail and succeed and how you can make yours last.* Simon & Schuster.

Prochaska, J., Norcross, J., DiClemente, C. (2007). *Changing for good: A revolutionary six-stage program for overcoming bad habits and moving your life positively forward.*

Travis, John MD, MPH. (2003). *The wellness workbook.* Wellness Associates.

Articles

Berkman, L.F. (1995). The role of social relations in health promotion. *Psychosomatic Medicine,* 57, 245-254.

Broadwell, S.D., Light, K.C. (1999). Family support, and cardiovascular responses in married couples during conflict and other interactions. *Int J Behav Med*, 6, 40-63.

Burdette, Bobbie. (2006). Excuses are valid.

Burdette, Bobbie. (2006). Learning and protecting modes.

Burdette, Bobbie. (2008). Authentic-Life Coaching.

Cohen, S., Doyle, W.J., Skoner, D.P., Rabin, B.S., Gwaltney, J.M. Jr (1997). Social ties and susceptibility to the common cold. *Journal of American Medical Association*, 277, 1940-44.

Gibb, Jack PhD. Defensive communication. *www.healthynet.com*.

Hein, Steve. Emotional intelligence. *www.eqi.org/eitoc.htm*.

McTaggart, Lynne. The power of intention. *Ode Magazine Online*, Issue 40.

Seeman, T.E., Berkman, L.F., Blazer, D., Rowe, J.W. (1994). Social ties and support and neuroendocrine functions: The MacArthur studies of successful aging. *Annals of Behavioral Medicine*, 16, 95-106.

Strohecker, James. (2006). A brief history of wellness.

Uchico, B.N., Cacioppo, J.T., Kiecolt-Glaser, J.K. (1996). The relationship between social support and physiological processes: A review with emphasis on underlying mechanism and implications for health. *Psychological Bulletin*, 119, 448-531.

ABOUT THE AUTHOR

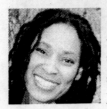 DR. MAIYSHA CLAIRBORNE IS AN American Board Certified family physician turned wellness and stress management coach. She is the founder of Mind Body Spirit Wellness Inc., where she focuses on helping clients achieve and maintain physical, emotional, and spiritual well-being.

Dr. Clairborne earned a BA in Psychology from Emory University. She completed her Medical Degree at Morehouse School of Medicine and finished her Family Medicine Residency at Florida Hospital in Orlando, FL. She completed her post-graduate training in acupuncture with The Academy of Pain Research Acupuncture and the International Academy of Medical Acupuncture.

Dr. Clairborne is the author of *Eat Your Disease Away*, which focuses on positive change through balance and nutrition. She has been featured as a wellness expert on the NBC40 Health Update, CW's *Focus Atlanta*, *Sacramento & Company*, and *Rx for Life*. She has also appeared on the nationally syndicated talk show *Daytime TV* and TLC's *Strange Addictions*.

Dr. Clairborne's expert articles appear in the *Derma-Scope Magazine*, *Disney Family Online*, *AOL Black Voices*, and the *Lovegevity* relationship column.

Dr. Maiysha Clairborne serves on the board of directors for the Georgia Coalition for Domestic Violence.

ALSO BY DR. CLAIRBORNE

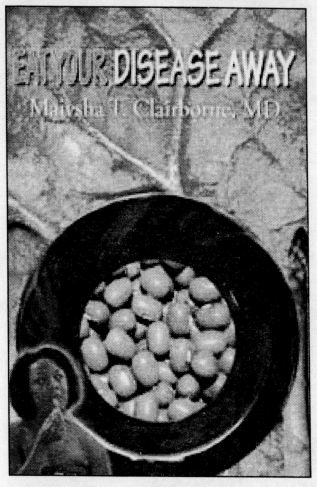

"Fix" Your Broken Metabolism, Fight Diseases, and
Lead a Happy and Healthy Life — with Ingredients
Hidden Right Inside Your Own Kitchen!

WWW.EATYOURDISEASEAWAY.COM

CONFERENCES, WORKSHOPS, RETREATS

DR. MAIYSHA CLAIRBORNE IS A SEASONED AND dynamic speaker who offers a variety of mind-body wellness programs worldwide. She thrives on creating extraordinary breakthroughs for individuals and groups through her interactive and results-oriented programs.

Contact Dr. Clairborne to have her

Δ   speak at your conference,

Δ   conduct a health & wellness workshop,

Δ   organize or take part in a retreat,

Δ   as an expert on a radio/TV interview.

WWW.MBSWELLNESS.ORG

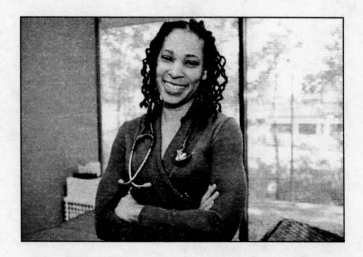